**DO NOT REMOVE
CARDS FROM POCKET**

Cocaine:
The Great White Plague

Cocaine:
The Great White Plague

Gabriel G. Nahas, M.D., Ph.D.

In Collaboration with Helene Peters

Foreword by Jacques Yves Cousteau

Paul S. Eriksson, *Publisher*

Middlebury, Vermont

Manufactured in the United States of America

10 9 8 7 6 5 4 3 2 1

Library of Congress Cataloging-in-Publication Data

Nahas, Gabriel G., 1920-
    Cocaine : the great white plague.

    Bibliography: p.
    Includes index.
    1. Cocaine habit—History. 2. Cocaine—History.
I. Title.
HV5810.N34 1989   362.29′8   89-16800
ISBN 0-8397-1700-8

To PRIDE and to parents everywhere.
To Marilyn and the family.
To future generations.

"There are a few clear areas in which we as a society must rise up united and express our intolerance, and the most obvious now is drugs. When the first cocaine was smuggled in on a ship, it may well have been a deadly bacterium, so much has it hurt the body and the soul of our country. There is much to be done and to be said, but take my word for it: this scourge will be stopped."

President George Bush
Inaugural address

Preface

This book, parts of which were first published in an abridged French version, *Les Guerres de la Cocaïne,* is a new, greatly enlarged volume. It incorporates the high points of studies and observations covering a period of twenty years in the field of drug dependence.

In writing the text I had the invaluable assistance of my sister. She deserves high praise for this and for a lifetime of collaboration with her grateful brother.

I present the personal testimony of a scientist. All the facts are drawn from verifiable primary sources. I have withheld identities of the individuals in the first part, "One Victim Among Many," but other principals are quoted from their public statements. I thank them for their unsolicited contributions.

I could not have written the book had I not participated in Captain Jacques Yves Cousteau's CALYPSO expedition to Peru, which was led by his son, Jean-Michel Cousteau. To father and son a friendly "Merci."

Although they are seldom mentioned in the text, the researchers working in my laboratory are entitled to a special expression of thanks. While I traveled throughout the Americas, they remained at home, diligently pursuing the basic research we had planned together, and which enabled us to understand more fully how cocaine interferes with normal chemical messages and affects vital heart and brain functions. A special salute goes to Renaud Trouvé and Colette Latour, whose studies took place under unusually difficult conditions with minimal financial support. Our work together led to the development of antidotes to the drug's lethal effects. This re-

viii Gabriel G. Nahas

search could not have been completed without the support of the Helen Clay Frick Foundation, to which I express heartfelt thanks.

This book does not conceal the gravity of the cocaine epidemic which is spreading through the Western world. The measures that must be taken are self-evident, dictated by common sense, history, and science, and clearly spelled out in our conclusions. It is our hope they will receive due consideration in the United States where the widespread usage of this drug has already resulted in devastating effects.

Gabriel Nahas

Contents

Foreword

The ability of man to disturb the ecology of the planet is matched by his propensity to pollute his own internal environment by using drugs of dependence. Among them, cocaine, extracted from the delicate leaf of a South American bush, is the most damaging, as clearly explained in this book. Cocaine, more than any addictive drug, impairs, at times, permanently, the fine brain mechanisms of "neurotransmission" essential for coherent, rational behavior.

The author is not only a most knowledgeable scientist, but he is also concerned about the safeguard of man. He seeks therefore to understand the social and biological factors likely to explain the causes of the present cocaine epidemic which has already taken on threatening dimensions in the Americas, and which is now spreading to Western Europe.

Few people — few governments — realize that this offensive of drugs (and specifically of cocaine) is simply an episode of a planned enterprise of destabilization of the Western world. We are living a war (undeclared but merciless) and in such times of national emergency only exceptional measures can overcome the threat. Only a strong public opinion can influence the leaders to organize seriously the defense of the Western culture.

Jacques Yves Cousteau

Cocaine:
The Great White Plague

I

ONE VICTIM AMONG MANY

1

Farid at the Hotel Pierre 1981

The phone rang in my laboratory at Columbia University: Hubert wanted to see me immediately at the Hotel Pierre. He couldn't talk but it was urgent. I agreed reluctantly. I was trying to finish a report, and a drive through Manhattan's evening traffic was a chore I could dispense with, even to oblige an old war buddy.

My yellow cab bounced along the pot-holed streets of Harlem as I wondered why Hubert had called me. He knew very well I wasn't practicing medicine, caught up as I had been for several years in projects on drugs whose casual use was on the rise everywhere.

Wearing a red carnation in his lapel and sporting a gold knob cane, my friend greeted me in the imposing hotel lobby. "It's on the fifth floor," he said as he took my arm.

We were alone in the elevator.

"Thanks for coming. I need your help with a customer who abused one of your favorite substances."

"Heroin?"

"No, coke."

"Could be just as serious. Any convulsions?"

"He's regaining consciousness. You'll see."

At the end of the corridor Hubert knocked on a double door. A statuesque young woman in a flimsy negligé greeted us. Her flowing black hair emphasized an olive complexion and dark almond-shaped eyes filled with distress.

"Come in, doctor."

I recognized the Middle-Eastern accent. We entered one of the most luxurious suites of the Pierre and stepped into a Louis XV sitting-room with richly upholstered gilt furniture, Farid, clad in a knee-length robe, was prostrate in an armchair. His swarthy Mediterranean features were further darkened by an unshaven beard and deep circles under his eyes. Appearing lost in a distant dream, he turned towards me.

"Doctor, I'm feeling fine."

"I believe he looks better," remarked Hubert.

I took his pulse. It was rapid but regular.

"When did he regain consciousness?"

"Just a few minutes ago," said the almond-eyed woman.

"There's nothing wrong with me," insisted Farid. "I'm just exhausted. You see, doctor, I work too hard."

He glanced at his companion. I had some difficulty understanding him. A strong nasal tone distorted his Middle-Eastern accent as if he suffered from a bad cold.

Hubert cut in:

"Look, you're talking to a well-known doctor and an old friend of mine. You can trust him."

"Hubert is right," I added. "I'm here to help you. Can I ask you a few questions? Your pulse is rapid and you just passed out."

Farid nodded wearily.

"Is it the first time you've passed out like this?"

"I think so. I don't really remember."

"And how long have you been on cocaine?"

"About three years."

"How did you get started?"

"In Los Angeles, with some friends in show business, at a party where everybody was sniffing coke. Anyway, it's relatively harmless. Nothing like heroin!"

"Nonsense; that's a myth. Obviously you're hooked on a very addictive drug which might kill you."

"You've got to be kidding," he replied irritably. "Where's the evidence? Can you prove it?"

"Certainly. A number of recent publications have reported deaths from cocaine overdose[1] confirming older observations."[2]

"Could I see them?"

"If you wish. I'll send them to you."

"No—it would take too long, and the mail isn't reliable. My chauffeur will drive you back to your lab and pick them up."

"Good idea," said Hubert.

"An unpleasant side-effect of coke," I went on, "is what it does to the mucous of the nose.[3] You speak with a strong nasal accent, but you don't have a cold."

"Yes, my nose has been bothering me."

"You should consult a specialist. You might have a perforation, a hole, in your septum."

I had touched a nerve because Farid asked me if I could recommend someone.

"I can, and if you want, I'll arrange an appointment."

"All right, as soon as possible. But I'm really more concerned about the deadly effects you mentioned. There are millions of coke users around and they seem quite well in control of their lives."

"Until they're trapped and become incurable addicts. . . ."

"Are you sure?" interrupted Farid. "Are you speaking from experience? Did you ever try cocaine?"

"Never. I wouldn't last very long if I tried all the toxic substances I study in my laboratory."

"Well, let me give you a little demonstration."

Hubert intervened:

"Farid, how about our deal? Shouldn't we take care of that first?"

"Don't worry, Hubert. I thought of it while you were gone."

He pulled a folded check from his pocket and handed it to Hubert, who slipped it in his wallet without looking at it.

"Now let me show you how harmless coke is," Farid said to me.

A scantily–clad woman who had been moving about the room brought him a delicate china plate. There were two parallel strips of white crystals on the plate. A crisp hundred-dollar bill rested on the edge. Farid rolled the bill into a thin straw and offered it to me.

"Come on," he said, "try it, at least once."

I declined, and so did Hubert, who exclaimed:

"For God's sake don't do it!"

Farid lowered his head, introduced the make-shift straw into a nostril and slowly inhaled the two lines of white powder. Eyes half-closed, face relaxed and smiling, he leaned his head on the back of his armchair.

"There!" he said. "I've just taken a good half–gram of coke and I feel perfectly lucid. I'm not dead either, as you can see!"

I was stunned. But my urge to intervene had to give way to professional detachment from a case over which I clearly had no control. I might just as well have been in my lab observing an experiment.

"May I take your pulse?"

He extended his wrist. Under my fingers I felt a quickening of the rhythm. In just two minutes his heartbeat had doubled and was at 140.

"Well, doctor, my heart is beating faster. I can feel it. But that happens also when I make love or play tennis. It's a sign of well-being and pleasure in a healthy male."

He then bolted out of his seat. The woman who had given him the cocaine and had sniffed some herself was laughing and trying to take off his robe.

"Don't," he said. "You're insatiable. Let me rest a little. Why don't you ask these gentlemen to oblige?"

Clearly, it was time for us to leave.

"Mr. Farid, I can't do anything more for you now. However, I must warn you: if you don't stop taking cocaine you'll be dead in two years."

"Listen to the doctor," urged Hubert.

"Che serà, serà," replied Farid. "My chauffeur will drive you back, and I'll be grateful if you'll give him the documents you promised me."

At the door of the suite, Farid's almond-eyed companion looked at me with infinite sadness. She was close to tears.

"Help us, doctor."

In the air-conditioned limousine with its tinted one-way vision windows, Hubert turned on the TV to catch the latest stock market transactions. He pulled out Farid's check, and after glancing at it, he handed it to me. Over an illegible signature an unsteady hand had scrawled, "Cash — one million dollars."

"You see," said Hubert. "Farid is one of the biggest gold brokers in the world. He can call Hong Kong, Paris, Rome, Riyadh, Sidney — you name it. Just on his word, he can close million–dollar deals in gold. An extraordinary mind."

"Maybe. . . . But if he keeps up this pace, he's a loser," I replied. "He'll die of an overdose."

Hubert looked at me with alarm.

"We've got to stop him, and I'm counting on you. After all these years you've spent studying drugs, shouldn't you have come up with a remedy by now?"

I caught the sarcasm.

"The trouble, Hubert, is that there's no medical treatment for coke addiction! There's only one cure: stop using the stuff. Sounds simple, but it isn't easy."

We reached the corner of 82nd street in a fashionable section of Manhattan. On the sidewalk, an elegantly-dressed lady was walking her poodle. Hubert shook my hand. "Thanks, Gaby. I'll call you tonight. Ciao."

The limousine glided out of the affluent neighborhood. I heard a click. The chauffeur had locked the doors. We had reached Harlem.

I have roamed through low-income districts in cities of the Middle East, almost overcome by the degradation and foul stench of human sewage. But somehow I felt safer in the slums of Cairo than on the streets of Harlem. Decay was everywhere: two-storied houses with torn shutters, plastic garbage bags piled on sidewalks, children playing on trash-filled curbs by gushing fire-hydrants. Partly-charred and boarded-up store-fronts punctuated the dismal scene.

Street lights shone on men loitering on sidewalks littered with broken glass. They were drinking beer or liquor out of brown-bagged bottles. At an intersection, behind another shiny limousine, dealers peddled drugs to passers-by.

Drugs have been around for decades in Harlem. It started in the twenties with marijuana, favored by jazz musicians, and was followed by heroin, with its aftermath of robberies, break-ins, vandalism, and the eventual decay of an area covering one-third of Manhattan.

Marijuana use spread to all social levels, including the affluent ones. Studies reported that in the United States ten percent of high school seniors were daily users of this so-called soft drug,[4] which sensitizes the brain to chemically-induced rewards and leads to more powerful drugs which kill — cocaine among others. For ten years I tried to convey this message to my colleagues in scientific and medical circles and to the general public. But I was preaching in the desert. After enjoying the pleasures of smoking marijuana, young Americans were discovering the delights of snorting cocaine, a drug that seemed made for them. Its use dispelled weariness and restored energy. I heard that the use of cocaine was increasing, especially among show people and in the business world. I had just witnessed a case myself. Why should I enter a new crusade against still another drug and its obvious destructive effects?

2

A Chewed-Up Nose

"Your friend Farid came to see me yesterday. Frankly, I've never examined a nasal cavity in worse shape: his septum is all chewed up."

I was listening to my colleague Harold, an ear, nose, and throat specialist, and munching a tasteless sandwich at the hospital cafeteria. Chicken salad or tuna fish? Who could tell?

"You mean that the partition in his nose is gone?" I asked.

Peering over his half-glasses with a perplexed air, he explained:

"You won't believe it. The cartilage is destroyed. When I introduced my speculum into his nose, I was afraid the nose would collapse because there wasn't any support left. The slightest pressure could flatten it out, and he'd have nostrils like a horse — what we call a saddle nose."

"Aren't septum perforations rather common among coke sniffers?"

"Yes, and they're well-described in the medical literature, especially in the older texts. They usually start no larger than a pinhead but can grow to the size of a dime. They used to be rare, but in the last two or three years I've been noticing more and more of them."

He shook his head.

"Farid's case beats anything I've seen so far. I don't have to tell you how cocaine interrupts the normal blood flow through the lining of the nose and after repeated contacts destroys this delicate tissue, baring the cartilage, which becomes infected and then perforated. In Farid's nose, all of the mucosa of the deeper nasal cavities are congested and inflamed."

"And you told him just that?"

"Why not? He seemed eager to know everything and understood perfectly well what I was saying; he's a very smart man."

"And what advice did you give him?"

"I prescribed antiseptic nosedrops and recommended he give up cocaine."

"Do you think he'll take that to heart?"

"Of course not! I made him think, though. He offered me a small fortune to insert a plastic partition in his nose!"

"Maybe he wanted a gold prosthesis, like what his dentist can give him."

"Come on! We don't have a reliable operational technique to treat even simple septum perforations! Let's face it; his case is hopeless."

Harold lifted his eyebrows:

"You know, this reminds me of something that happened recently to a lovely actress, the picture of innocence with an angel face and an exquisite nose. She had a perforated septum and desperately begged me to do something. I sent her to Andy, our top plastic surgeon, who performed a graft of mucosa to cover the perforation, since cartilage can't be grafted. The operation was a success."

"You see! There really are some solutions."

"Yes—only our young beauty returned to her old ways and pretty soon an infection developed around the graft and the hole reappeared bigger than ever! So she sued Andy, me, and the hospital for malpractice."

"She must have lost her case. After all, cocaine is a controlled substance."

"She did lose it—barely. The jury and the judge listened to her with great sympathy. Her lawyer even called a witness, a psychiatrist, who testified that cocaine was a harmless recreational drug and that it is unfair to penalize its users."

"You had your own expert, too, I assume."

"Of course. A pharmacologist, like you. He gave a slide presentation demonstrating the effect of the drug on the mucosa, which becomes as white as the cocaine powder. The tightening of the capillaries stops the blood flow entirely. You can cut right into the mucosa and you won't see a drop of blood. Amazing. To return to your friend, he doesn't seem to want to stop."

"I gave him quite a scare when I told him he'd be dead in

two years if he didn't quit. I sent him a recent article from
J.A.M.A.[1] describing seventy well-documented cases of death
by cocaine overdose. Still, at this point he's sniffing large
quantities—between five and fifteen grams a day."

"He must be spending a mint on his habit, with the
running price of coke powder at two hundred dollars a gram!
Of course, you realize we're paying only ten dollars a gram
when we buy it for use as a topical anaesthetic for our patients."

"You can see why some of our colleagues are tempted to
take advantage of those bargain prices for their private needs.
But how about Farid? With his mucosa practically shot, its
capacity to absorb the drug must be quite restricted."

"Considerably so," concurred Harold, "and that accounts
for his enormous consumption. But although very small
amounts of the drug are reaching his blood vessels, they keep
destroying the lining of his nose."

"That's why he might be starting shooting the stuff or,
worse, smoking it—the latest fad."

"You're kidding! Smoking cocaine?" Harold appeared be-
mused.

"Sure. But, mind you, it's not the chloride salt of cocaine
which is used for anesthesia. That would be destroyed by the
heat of a cigarette. What is smoked is a "cocaine base," easily
made by chemical manipulation of the cocaine chloride. In this
basic form, it vaporizes when smoked and is picked up by the
blood in the lung. Very high concentrations of the drug reach
the brain."

"Madness, complete madness," Harold muttered.

I agreed, but my thoughts kept returning to the man at
the Hotel Pierre. Hubert had called to tell me Farid was
impressed by the documents I sent him and, encouraged by
Yasmine, his almond-eyed companion, he was resolved to give
up cocaine. Moreover, he intended to leave New York and
settle in Paris where the temptation to use drugs would be less.

Threatened with death, Farid, at least, had granted himself a reprieve.

3

From Cocaine to Vitamins

A week later Hubert phoned me again. He sounded worried and asked me to get in touch immediately with the American Hospital in Paris. Farid had been taken to the intensive care unit there.

"I've got to know if he's going to make it. The doctors won't talk to me about his condition. But I'm sure they'll discuss it with a colleague like you."

An important financial transaction could turn sour for my friend if something happened to Farid. I felt obliged to help, although I would have preferred to forget the whole affair.

I reached one of the doctors at the hospital where Farid had been admitted the day before in a deep coma interrupted by convulsions. He was on an artificial respirator and on Valium while several liters of salt solution were being pumped into his system. He was improving and would shortly be off the respirator. He was expected to regain consciousness any time.

"And what is your diagnosis?"

"It's hard to tell. Some sort of poisoning seems likely, but all the toxicological tests are negative."

"Did you test for cocaine?"

"No only for opiates, barbiturates and amphetamines, too."

I informed the Paris doctor that Farid was seriously hooked on coke. A look at his nasal cavities would be proof enough. My suggestion was to send him to a rehabilitation center as soon as he was released.

"You mean to a psychiatric clinic?" inquired the doctor.

"No, rather to a special drug-free rehabilitation center, like the one run by Le Patriarche."

"By whom, did you say?"

"Le Patriache, Lucien Engelmayer."[1]

"Never heard of him, but I'll make a note of your recommendation."

I thanked him and left my number so Farid could call me.

At daybreak the next morning, an enraged Farid was on the line. He hadn't bothered to check the time differential before calling. He blurted out angrily:

"I . . . I feel just fine. You just mind your own business."

"Farid, try to understand. . . . "

"Leave me alone. I don't need a detoxification treatment, or any of your psychiatrists and all their malarkey."

"Farid, if you don't listen to me, you're going to kill yourself."

He hung up. That morning I briefed Hubert on his friend's health.

"He's alive," I told him, "but surely not for long. He just can't stay away from his drug. In my lingo we call it compulsive behavior."

"Such an intelligent guy," lamented Hubert. "I can't understand what's going on."

"You've got to realize that intelligence has very little to do with the control of our emotions, with *l'amour*. And Farid has fallen in love with cocaine."

"Why are you so hard on Farid? He's a terrific guy, very capable and well worth saving. If you knew how useful he is to us on Wall Street!"

"No doubt, but our hands are tied if he doesn't cooperate."

"Well, in any case, I'm not giving up — yet. I know his family and friends. Maybe they can help."

"You mean his lovely companion with the big sad eyes?"

"Ah, you noticed her, too. Yes, I was thinking of her, of course, but also of Farid's brother who's a sort of bodyguard to him."

I wished Hubert good luck and assured him he could count on my support.

A month went by. Then I was in Paris and gave Farid a call. Hubert had given me a message for him. The nasal voice attempted to sound cordial and I was invited to stop by his apartment that evening.

Farid lived in a plush apartment building on the Avenue Montaigne, a tree-lined street, one of the most select in Paris.

A suspicious doorman, after grilling me on my identity, announced my visit. He then escorted me to the third floor, where a tall, dark young man met me.

"Come in, please." He ushered me inside and shot the three bolts to secure the heavy door.

"I'm Farid's brother," he announced with some pride.

In the spacious, elegantly–furnished sitting room, the master of the house greeted me. His companion was at his side.

"It's very kind of you to bring Hubert's message in person."

He slipped Hubert's letter into his pocket and added: "How's old Hubert doing?" The nasal tones were more controlled. The relaxed features expressed a serenity I hadn't seen before.

"He's fine, only he's very concerned about your health!" Farid shook his head.

"Do me a favor. Tell him to stop worrying about me, won't you?"

"Does that mean you're off cocaine?" I asked abruptly.

Farid affected a casual tone:

"Yes, since I've been back in Paris and after your last phone call. I've made up my mind not to return to New York. Over there everybody's into drugs. There's no way you can get away."

"Come on, Farid, aren't you exaggerating a little?"

"Maybe it's different in your scientific and medical circles, although I happen to know plenty of your colleagues who get regularly high on coke—they've got easy access to it."

I was indeed aware that more and more doctors were using drugs. Things had reached such a pass that recently professional committees had been appointed by medical associations to ensure that state regulations were being followed and to keep track of physicians who abused their privileges by prescribing large quantities of restricted drugs for their own use.

"On the other hand," continued Farid, "businessmen and women, brokers, bankers, lawyers, showbiz people do drugs. It's as routine as smoking tobacco or taking a drink. You'll find drugs at social gatherings and any time people close a business deal."

"In that case, you certainly made the right move when you decided not to return to the States."

"I'm thinking of staying here for good because I can run my business from Paris just as well. The time-zone situation keeps me up at night to follow the Big Board on Wall Street, but I can deal with that."

His companion smiled approvingly. I congratulated him on his decision and asked if I could do anything for him.

"To be honest, doctor, I could use something to help me stay off coke when I feel depressed, anxious, or restless. At this point, I'm following my dear mother's advice. I'm very much into vitamins."

"Which ones?"

"All of them. Here—take a look."

Farid opened a sideboard filled with silver, china, and crystal. On the middle shelf flasks and jars were lined up in neat rows. I read a few labels at random: they listed various vitamin and mineral contents.

"And which ones do you take?"

"Oh, I just dig in. I've read the labels and they're all pretty much the same."

"How many tablets do you take?"

"About ten a day."

One of my colleagues once noted jokingly that the main effect of vitamins, which tend to be eliminated quickly through the kidneys, is to produce a high-priced ordinary body fluid. Vitamins could not do much to dissipate his craving for cocaine.

"I'm quite sure," continued Farid, "that these products are useful and that they seem to strengthen me. But I need something to shake off the weariness and the anguish that get to me."

Farid was admitting he suffered from withdrawal symptoms. They are different from those induced by heroin. Those present visible signs of mental and physical distress. Farid's were subtler and deeper manifestations, not unlike the haunting memories left by the loss of a dear one.

"I'm sorry, but you can't break an addiction to a mind-stimulating substance like cocaine by turning to another product that does the same thing! You can't stop getting drunk on red wine by drinking white wine."

"Then what's the answer?" Farid looked at me intently.

"There's only one way: change your life habits."

I had in mind the rehabilitation centers known as "therapeutic communities," where former addicts attempt to rebuild their lives in a drug-free environment.

"You can't go it alone," I continued. "You need the support of a group of people as determined as you are to shake off the drug habit."

Farid's face was glum. His companion drew closer to him and put her hand on his shoulder.

"You should listen to the doctor," she said.

"Oh, I'm listening to him all right," Farid retorted testily.

"I should add, in all fairness, that getting hooked on cocaine is the worst addiction of all. To kick the habit, you've got to stay away from the stuff for a long time and relearn how to live without it."

"How do you do that?"

"By joining a group dedicated to this kind of rehabilitation. Because we're talking rehabilitation, not treatment. For a while you'd lead a kind of communal life. And Yasmine could even be with you. If you're ready to take this step, I'll tell you more about the program."

"And how long would I have to stay at the center?"

"Six months at least,"

Farid shrugged his shoulders impatiently.

"You're not serious," he scoffed. "I've got my occupation, my business. I could stay away a week maybe two, at most. More is out of the question."

He shook his head vigorously as Yasmine looked on sadly. Farid was not ready for the only move that might save him from a relapse, a relapse that could be fatal.

"I understand your hesitation. If you change your mind, here's a phone number you can call any time."

I gave him the number of Le Patriarche, who could be reached twenty-four hours a day.

"Thank you, but I'm sure I won't need it. By the way, Hubert will be in Paris tomorrow. Why don't you join us for diner at the Pavillon de l'Elysée around 8:30?"

I accepted the invitation.

"Until then, think about my suggestion. We can talk more about it."

Farid made a vague gesture. I knew he was unable to lead a calm and sedentary life for very long. The support of his companion's love and his family's devotion would not be enough. The obsessive memory of the pleasures made readily available by the most stimulating of all drugs was imprinted in his brain and still too fresh.

In the side alley, in front of the building, a white Rolls Royce was parked under the impassive gaze of the doorman. Farid's brother was engaged in a heated exchange with the chauffeur.

I heard the brother shout: "I've already told you he isn't here!"

4

The Curtain Falls

I lingered over coffee with Hubert, Farid, and Yasmine at the Pavillon Elysée. On this beautiful June evening the temperature was so mild and the breeze so caressing that the big awning over the outdoor summer restaurant had been rolled back and we sat under the stars.

Farid seemed gloomier than usual and the eyes of his companion a little sadder. Her lovely face brightened only when Hubert, always one to enliven a conversation, told a funny story.

It was about a farmer who saw a penguin splashing in his pond. The local school-teacher, consulted on the matter, advised the farmer to take the bird to the zoo, where it probably had come from. A week later the penguin was still wading among the ducks in the farmer's pond. "Well, you didn't take him to the zoo, I see," said the school-teacher. "You betcha I did," replied the farmer, "and she enjoyed herself very much. This Saturday, I'm taking her to the ball game."

Before leaving the restaurant I had a chance to talk for a minute to Yasmine and ask her if Farid had thought about treatment at one of Le Patriarche's rehabilitation centers. Fear flashed through her eyes. She shook her head.

"Please don't even mention it to him."

Before we parted I noticed, parked at a short distance from the restaurant, the same white Rolls Royce that had been stationed the other night in front of Farid's apartment house.

Hubert and I were strolling under the chestnut trees of the Avenue Gabriel on our way to his hotel.

"Don't you think," remarked Hubert, as we were passing in front of the American Embassy, "that our friend has improved and that his stay in Paris agrees with him?"

Knowing the craving induced by cocaine, I doubted Farid's chances to break his addiction by himself. To succeed he had to accept the discipline of a new life-style which he could not achieve without the extended support of a rehabilitation community.

"Sorry, Hubert. I don't want to play Cassandra, but Farid is still very vulnerable, even in Paris. Although this isn't New York, there's a thriving cocaine trade among some of the very rich guys coming from the oil states of the Gulf and now jet-setting all over Europe. Farid knows a lot of them."

"You mean he'll go back to coke?"

"It's more than likely."

"And you can't do anything about it?"

"No, I can't force him to follow the only treatment that will save him. You've got to realize that a drug addict is a lot like a character out of a Greek tragedy, stricken by a blind fate.

"Come on, leave literature out of this."

"This isn't literature, Hubert. It's just a way of telling you I'm powerless, and so is medicine."

"Don't go to all that trouble! I've got to know if there's any risk in doing business with Farid."

"As far as I'm concerned, I don't have the slightest doubt! I wouldn't trust him with a dime."

I left Hubert at the Place de la Concorde in front of the Hotel Crillon, where cars swept in circles around the brightly lit Luxor obelisk. Encountering only a few pedestrians at that late hour, I walked slowly to my apartment, deep in thought. To my knowledge, France is the only country in the world where penal law may punish anyone who does not assist a person whose life is in jeopardy.[1] I found myself breaking that law because of a society of tolerance that had trivialized drug use in the name of freedom of choice and the individual's right to self-destruction.

I never saw Farid again. Shortly after our last meeting he was arrested by the French Narcotics Brigade for cocaine traffic. Released on $500,000 bond, he jumped bail and flew to Colombia. Hubert told me of his death in Bogotá, later that Fall. His naked and bruised body was found by a maid in the ransacked room of a luxury hotel. Nobody had claimed the body. Neither the police nor the autopsy could clearly establish the cause of death. It was probably a drug overdose, perhaps the fruit of infighting among cocaine warlords.

Farid's death came as no surprise to me, but I had not expected such a sordid end. I was more outraged than hurt. This absurd and useless killing was not the only one that could be attributed to cocaine. The victims of cocaine were numbered in the hundreds, even thousands, since drug traffic and use was increasing year after year. Every day, doctors must resign themselves to witnessing the deaths of incurably-ill patients despite dedicated and intense efforts to heal them by drawing on the growing medical resources of the late twentieth century. Unfortunately, there is no medication that can cure the suicidal behavior of the addict whose brain has been poisoned by cocaine. Should we then look on powerless, as human beings self-destruct in our so-called age of progress? For my part, I reject such a surrender. At the time the curtain fell on Farid's life I did not suspect that through the force of circumstances I was about to enter a long and difficult combat.

5

A Trial in Newark and Cement Boots

Shortly after Farid's death in the fall of 1981, I was contacted by the district attorney of the City of Newark. He had seen one of my articles in the "United Nations Bulletin on Narcotics" where I classified cocaine as an addictive and dangerous drug.[1]

"You have the professional qualifications," he told me over the phone, "to appear in court as an expert for the prosecution. Would you agree to testify in a case of cocaine traffic?"

I felt little inclination to oblige. The memory of lengthy and exhausting sessions where I was called to take the stand at trials involving marijuana dealers did not encourage me to repeat the experience.

"But the dangers of cocaine are evident," I told him. "It's a killer drug and it induces a greater dependency than heroin. We have known that for a hundred years."

"That's your opinion, doctor. But I have in front of me the testimony of a witness for the defense, a Harvard professor, who declares, and I quote: 'Cocaine is a recreational drug that can be used, as it frequently is, without causing significant physiological alterations.' "

This sounded like my Harvard colleague Lester Grinspoon whom I had faced on various occasions where he testified that marijuana was a drug much less dangerous to health than alcohol or tobacco, that should therefore be legalized.[2] And now Grinspoon — if it was he — was underplaying the dangers of "recreational use" of "moderate" doses of cocaine.[3]

"Yes, sir, some psychiatrists hold those views; but most pharmacologists don't agree."

"And that's why I'm asking you to testify."

"But you have two medical schools at your doorstep, one in Newark, the other at Rutgers. My colleagues in pharmacology could testify as well as I. Have you contacted any of them?"

A brief silence followed. Then the district attorney went on, speaking carefully:

"Well—they're not free at trial-time. One is tied up with his courses and another will be out of town. They also tell me that they don't consider themselves competent enough, since they haven't personally conducted studies on the drug."

"I'm somewhat in the same situation. I'm directing research projects, preparing lectures, and, in addition, getting ready for a trip to Paris next week. Furthermore, I haven't conducted my own experiments on the toxicity of that drug. It's already been so firmly established."

"Doctor, we can select a date that fits your schedule."

The district attorney's insistence seemed to indicate that my New Jersey colleagues were not willing to testify.

"But why is my testimony so important to you?"

"Not to me, Doctor. Let me explain the situation. In New Jersey, as in the rest of the U.S., cocaine is classified, with opiates, as a narcotic, a drug inducing a swift and dangerous dependency. Any non-medical use is punished by law, and traffic in narcotics calls for ten to fifteen years in jail. In the present case the accused was caught with over ten pounds of cocaine in his possession, which could get him a fifteen–year prison sentence without parole. The defense lawyer is challenging the state laws by arguing that cocaine is not a narcotic like heroin and that it's less dangerous than amphetamines.[4] The penalty for illegal traffic in amphetamines, which have a wider medical use than cocaine, is a three to five year prison sentence. Finally, the defense claims that cocaine usage is not dangerous to consumers or to society and therefore that our cocaine state laws are antiquated, unfair and unsupported by modern scientific data."

"In other words, the defense is challenging narcotics laws which, those lawyers say, are unjustly penalizing citizens instead of protecting society."

"Exactly. And if the judge accepts these arguments, the trial will be delayed until a decision is reached by an appellate court. A judgment favorable to the accused could establish a precedent we want to avoid."

Once more, I was surprised at the pliability of Anglo-Saxon common law. When a law no longer suits the citizenry, it is modified to adjust to current trends. I felt uncomfortable with this type of judicial practice. For me, the case of cocaine was clear: it was an extremely dangerous substance and any legalistic sophistry that attempted to make it socially acceptable was pure fallacy which should be countered with unequivocal medical and scientific arguments. Furthermore, Farid's case was still fresh in my mind.

"All right, I'll testify," I agreed, albeit reluctantly.

The police car that drove me to the courthouse was approaching Newark, the most dilapidated industrial port on the Eastern seaboard. The low-income sectors of town were not unlike parts of Harlem: garbage-littered crumbling sidewalks where a garish crowd sauntered in front of run-down housing.

"On this street," confided my driver, "you can buy any kind of drug, you name it: marijuana, hash, cocaine, heroin, barbiturates,[5] L.S.D.[6] We cleaned it up last month. We put forty-five pushers behind bars and seized a pile of dope. And today we're back where we started: the dealers are all over, they're often the same guys, out on parole, peddling their stuff." He shook his head. "You can't just let it take over the country. You've got to do something."

The courtroom was packed. The accused, a man in his thirties, was seated in the front row next to his wife and two children. After I took the oath and gave my name and credentials, the judge asked me to describe the effects of cocaine. My slide presentation followed the didactic format requested by the prosecutor. First I defined the drug, both in legal and in pharmacological terms. For the legislator, "a narcotic" is a substance which impairs behavior and induces a dependency harmful to man and society. In this legal sense, cocaine is classified with other drugs which produce dependency, such as cannabis or opiates, and are restricted, by international agreement, to medical and scientific uses. However, for the pharmacologist cocaine is a stimulant, quite different from opiates which are sedatives. The classification of cocaine as a narcotic has, therefore, a strictly legal and operational basis. I proceeded to describe the pleasure-inducing and tonic properties of cocaine, which dispel weariness, clear the mind, stimulate mental activity, and confer a feeling of quiet dominance and serene power. The urge to repeat a pleasant experience more and more frequently appears shortly after taking cocaine, showing the dark side of the coin: as consumption increases, euphoria is followed by depression and anxiety. Furthermore, sniffing may damage the nose so severely that the user will resort to intravenous injections. At this stage, psychic disorders set in, which may eventually lead to criminal violence, hallucinations such as the sensation of insects crawling under the skin, and even suicide. Hospitalization in a psychiatric unit becomes necessary. Injections may cause death by cardiac failure or convulsions.

"Are injections the only cause of death?" inquired the judge.

"No, the medical literature reports a number of lethal cases[7] occurring after sniffing cocaine or applying it to the nasal mucosa for purposes of local anesthesia."

In conclusion, I emphasized the obsessional character of the self-administration process for the addict whose unique goal in life becomes finding and consuming the drug.

To illustrate the compulsive behavior induced by cocaine, in 1969 I projected a short film produced by the University of Michigan scientists Deneau and Yanagita under the direction of the famous pharmacologist, Professor Maurice Seevers.[8] The film shows a monkey harnessed with a special apparatus that allows him complete freedom in his cage and lets him inject various substances into his veins by pressing on a lever. The animal selects exclusively dependency–producing drugs: opiates, amphetamines, and cocaine, ignoring other choices, such as aspirin or penicillin. Furthermore, in a unique pattern, the animal self-injects cocaine in such quantities that he dies within three weeks. The most dramatic sequence of the film shows the frenzied animal pressing the lever while going into convulsions. The moment he recovers, he returns, still shaking, to his lever for a new dose.

After my testimony, the defense lawyer asked me abruptly if I would call cocaine a "narcotic."

"Not from a strictly pharmacological point of view," I replied, "but legally, yes."

The judge straightened himself in his chair.

"The doctor," he said to the defense attorney, "did explain that distinction very clearly. No further explanation is necessary."

Disappointed, the lawyer pursued his line of questioning:

"Is cocaine as dangerous and toxic as amphetamines?"

"Absolutely. As I mentioned earlier, cocaine use can

cause accidents as serious as those due to amphetamines and can lead to death by overdose, or to criminal and self-destructive behavior."

"Certain researchers have opposing views," he continued, "and I could quote Professors Grinspoon[9] and Norman Zinberg[10] and Dr. Andrew Weil,[11] all from Harvard."

"My colleagues[12] refer only to users who sniff small amounts of cocaine, sometimes mixed with powdered sugar. Frequent injections into the veins or under the skin often induce severe disorders described in the scientific and medical exhibits which were turned over to the state as part of my testimony."

"Does cocaine produce a physical dependency?"

"It does in the form of biochemical, therefore physical, alterations of the brain."

"Such as?"

"Important modifications of adrenalin–like substances produced in brain cells. These substances control the coherent and continuous transmission of signals throughout the brain circuits."

"Hasn't it been established, however, that cocaine doesn't create a real dependency, as heroin does, with withdrawal symptoms?"

"Cocaine, which is chemically different from heroin or the opiates, also has different mechanisms of action on the brain. Cocaine does not induce withdrawal symptoms similar to those that occur after abstinence from opiates. However, the interruption of cocaine use produces its specific withdrawal symptoms such as depression, anxiety, and exhaustion."

"But many scientists, including Professor Charles Schuster from the University of Chicago, characterize cocaine dependency as purely psychological in nature. Your testimony is in complete disagreement with his!"

I had been sent Schuster's testimony,[13] given a few months earlier before the Appellate Court of the State of Illinois in a case similar to the one tried in Newark. Dr. Schuster, a psychologist, had administered limited amounts of cocaine to volunteer cocaine addicts, and reported the following: "Under the experimental conditions of my laboratory, the only psychological changes observed are increases in friendly euphoria and happiness. . . . Frequency of paranoia is very low. . . . There are no cardiac abnormalities expect for a heart rate increase. . . . Frequency of aggressive behavior is very low." He went on to report he had not seen physical symptoms or withdrawal symptoms.

I could well understand the bewilderment of the defense lawyer confronted with testimonies as conflicting as Schuster's and my own!

I went on expressing my own viewpoint which, I remained convinced, was closer to pharmacological reality:

"Scientists differ — and in this case my colleagues are using an obsolete terminology which does not take into account recent scientific discoveries. Interruption of cocaine use produces residual disorder symptoms in cerebral activity, apathy, depression, and sleeping disorders with abnormal brain wave patterns which may last for weeks."

"I have no more questions, your Honor."

Having run out of arguments, the lawyer returned to his seat.

The judge pounded his gavel and the audience rose. Addressing the prosecutors and defense lawyers, he stated that, after a thorough examination of all the evidence, he would render his decision at a later date.

The gavel pounded the desk once more. "The court is adjourned."

The judge shook my hand and walked into his adjoining chambers. As I passed by the defendant, our eyes met and I felt his glare of hatred. Should the present scheduling for a cocaine offense be upheld, he might receive the maximum sentence — fifteen years in jail. I was aware that my vocation as a physician was to care for the sick, not to condemn others or be a party to their condemnation. Why should I become entangled in the judicial process incumbent upon our courts? "Judge not that ye be not judged,"[14] declared the Scriptures that had shaped my thinking as a youth. If some colleagues resented my position so strongly, was it that they felt I was overstepping my role as a physician?

Nevertheless, a few hundred milligrams of cocaine can kill a man. Those ten pounds of cocaine, some five million milligrams, he had when he was arrested could cause the death of several users and start many others on the path of a most enslaving addiction while bringing wealth to an anonymous murderer.

That evening when I returned to my laboratory, everyone

had left. I was in a reflective mood. I sat at my littered desk, wondering why prominent American psychiatrists and intellectuals still refused to recognize the damaging effects of cocaine and its addictive nature. The answer to this question came to my mind after glancing at the three books still opened on my desk and which I had studied to prepare for my testimony at the Newark trail. They were the *Cocaine Papers* of Sigmund Freud,[15] *Phantastica* by Ludwig Lewin,[16] and *Der Kocainismus* by Hans Maier.[17] These books documented the acrimonious debate which had pitted two leading physicians, a pharmacologist and a psychiatrist, against Freud one hundred years ago. Before he became a renowned psychoanalyst, Freud had endorsed the use of cocaine in medicine because he attributed safety and great healing powers to it. The controversy between these men bore a striking resemblance to the opposing parties at the Newark trial.

The phone rang. I heard a deep voice. "You deserve cement boots and you'll get 'em." I hung up wearily. I had received similar unpleasant calls some ten years before when I was exposing the health hazards of hashish and marijuana use, adding fuel to a controversy which was still lingering. Somehow, this time, I felt I was on the verge of becoming involved in a more critical debate. How could I best prepare for the fight that lay ahead? By a critical analysis of the older literature, which is neglected by today's psychiatrists, and then by proceeding with new experimental studies of the addictive properties of cocaine.

To pursue that course, I now turn to the past in order to discuss some episodes from the cocaine wars and analyze the literature in which they appear. This will throw much-needed light on today's debates and also permit me to lay out a chart for a course of new experimental research on cocaine.

II

THE GREAT COCAINE CONTROVERSY:
FROM THE 1880'S TO THE 1920'S

6

Freud's Praise of Cocaine

In 1884 Sigmund Freud had completed his medical studies in Vienna and was working as an assistant in the University Laboratory of Experimental Medicine where he studied the pathology of the nervous system. He was twenty-eight years old. Freud, like any other ambitious young scientist, was looking for a project that would lead to a major discovery and from there to fame in the medical world, public recognition, and, eventually, financial affluence. The modest position at the University Laboratory was a stepping stone which would, after the publication of an original research contribution, allow him to become a "Privat Dozent," the first rank of the tenured faculty, and assure him a promising career at the famed University of Vienna. He would then at last be able to marry his fiancée, Martha Bernays, to whom he had already been engaged for three years.

At the time, there was a great deal of discussion in Viennese medical circles about cocaine. A few doctors in Europe, and more still in the United States, praised its properties. This substance, extracted from the leaves of the shrub "Coca Erythroxylon," had been identified by two German chemists from the University of Göttingen, Albert Nieman and William Lossen,[1] some twenty years earlier. Freud was especially impressed by the reports of a Bavarian Army doctor, Theodore Aschenbrandt,[2] who had fed cocaine to mountain artillery men and observed beneficial and stimulating effects of that drug on soldiers exposed to inclement weather and exhausting climbs. Reports coming from the United States hailed cocaine as an effective treatment for morphine addiction. Was this a new miracle drug? After testing its effects on himself, Freud became convinced it was just that and referred to it as a "magical" substance which boosted his working capacity while awakening pleasure and motivation, especially when he felt tired or in a slump. He even sent some to his fiancée, with the promise that this white powder would "give her energy and rosy cheeks."[3] After further successful experiments on himself, Freud prescribed cocaine to his best friend, the physiologist Ernst von Fleishl. A charming and exceedingly brilliant man, von Fleishl had become a morphine addict as a result of daily self-injections to relieve sharp pains caused by the amputation of a thumb. "Von Fleishl," Freud tells us, "seized on the new drug with the desperation of a drowning man." In July, 1884, on the strength of his preliminary observations, Freud published his article *Uber Coca*[4] (*On Coca*), which he dedicated to Martha as "a hymn in praise of that magical substance." The scope of the survey caused quite a stir in the medical world. While Freud briefly mentions his own limited experience with the drug, he devotes most of his paper to a review of all the available literature on coca which could be found in the library of the Vienna Medical School.

To begin with, Freud describes the coca tree, a five-foot bush similar to a hawthorn shrub, grown on the western slopes of the Andes at altitudes of three to six thousand feet over an area from Peru to Bolivia in the heart of the tropics. The French botanist Jussieu[5] recorded the plant's features and placed it in the Erythroxylon genus. J. B. Lamarck[6] gave it the name Erythroxylon Coca in his Encyclopédie Méthodique Botanique.

"Its small and pretty oval leaves constitute an indispensable food for some ten million people," says Freud.

> The bush yields small white flowers on each of its two or three lateral stems. Seeds or cuttings are planted and later transplanted. The first crop can be harvested within eighteen months. A coca bush yields two to five crops per year and has a life of thirty to forty years! The leaves are ripe when their stems snap at a light touch. They are dried in the sun or in an oven and are ready for consumption.[7]

Freud then covers the history and use of coca in Peru, its country of origin. According to legend, the divine Manco Capac,

> sent by his father the God Sun, came down, at the dawn of time, from the boulders of Lake Titicaca, to bring the gift of light to the poor. . . . He taught them the story of the gods, the practice of daily crafts, and he gave them coca, the sacred plant

which feeds the hungry, strengthens the weak and allows them to forget their misery. Coca leaves were offered in sacrifice to the gods, they were chewed during religious ceremonies and were even placed in the mouths of the dead to insure their welcome in the other world. . . .

But the Spanish Conquistadores did not believe in the extraordinary virtues of the plant. Rather continues Freud,

They saw in it a device of the devil because of the important part it played in the religious ceremonies of the defeated people. A council of Spanish officials met in Lima and went so far as to prohibit its consumption, which was considered a pagan custom and a sin. However, the new Spanish rulers changed their minds as soon as they noticed that without coca the Indians were unable to perform the heavy tasks assigned to them in the mines. From then on, three to four times a day, they distributed coca leaves to the workers and granted them short pauses during which they chewed the leaves they were so fond of. Nowadays, an Indian always carries a little bag of coca leaves and a flask filled with ashes or chalky soil. The Indian chews the leaves into a ball and wedges it between the gum and the cheek, poking it at regular intervals with a needle dipped in the ash.[8]

The Indian consumes this "food" from youth throughout his life. He increases his usual dose when he covers long distances, takes a woman, or has to muster his strength to engage in a sustained activity.

Reports by contemporary explorers describe how the Indians, under the influence of coca, could withstand unusual stress and perform superhuman tasks without eating. "Indians who consume coca are able to walk for hundreds of hours and run as fast as horses without showing any signs of fatigue." Freud even quotes from the memories of Von Tschudi[9] whose servant,

a half-breed, performed, during five days and five nights in a row, deep excavations without sleeping more than two hours at night or eating anything but coca . . . After he finished his work, he ran for two days alongside Tschudi's mule and declared he would readily repeat the same work if he were supplied with enough coca. This sixty-two year old man had never been sick.

The ability of coca users to withstand lack of food for extended periods without suffering any physiological damage seems to have made a considerable impression on Freud, who accepts reports claiming that "in some parts of Peru the people often eat nothing for several days: they chew coca and work continuously."

Such anecdotal accounts are never questioned by Freud, who will, however, criticize diverging views claiming that "the effect of coca is purely imaginary and that the natives are capable of accomplishing the same tasks without coca, through practice and coercion." He quotes but one dissident voice, that of his compatriot Poepigg.[10] This author of "many slanderous statements on coca" draws "a frightening picture of the physical and intellectual degradation of the Indians, an inevitable consequence of coca use." Freud rejects Poepigg's interpretation:

> As early as the 17th Century, Jesuits and Spanish doctors, such as Father Julian[11] and Dr. Monardes,[12] upon their return from Peru, praised the astonishing virtues of the plant that appeases hunger and fatigue. All the other observers agree that a moderate consumption of coca is more favorable than harmful and that "coqueiros" die at an advanced age.

In presenting these anecdotal reports, Freud gave scant attention of the recommendations of Claude Bernard[13] in his "Introduction to the Study of Experimental Medicine," published in 1865. "We must not believe in our observations and our theories without the support of an experimental inventory. If one believes too much," says Bernard, "the mind is bound and narrowed by the effects of its own reasoning; it no longer enjoys freedom of action and therefore lacks the initiative of those who can rid themselves of a blind faith in theories, which is nothing but scientific superstition." Basic notions of physiology, as taught then by Bernard and his pupils, should have tempered Freud's enthusiasm for cocaine. He could have wondered how a substance devoid of caloric value could increase muscular activity while the food input which generates the energy necessary for work was decreased. The observations of contemporary European researchers are, on the whole, quite disappointing to Freud when weighed against the explorers' reports on Peru. For example, according to a report from a British physiology laboratory, experiments meant to demonstrate the energizing effect of cocaine "produced no results whatsoever," and thereafter researchers stopped studying coca in England.

Experimental observations do not impress Freud. For him the sparing effect "of coca on the quantity of food needed for a given energy output" seems scientifically acceptable. "An organism under the influence of a dose of cocaine, even a small one," he tells us, "can draw from the substance a larger amount of vital strength than without the drug and this strength can be converted into work. Under the influence of cocaine an organism has a lower metabolism and needs less food to perform a prolonged task." This hypothesis, according to Freud, "does not necessarily contradict the law of conservation of energy." Indeed, Freud claims, if an energy output resulting from work requires a caloric intake provided normally by food, it is possible to decrease this caloric intake by "appropriate measures."

Freud seems to endow cocaine with a magical sparing factor that he cannot explain although he is aware of experiments by Claude Bernard[14] which invalidate his thesis. Bernard studied loss of weight among animals deprived of food and compared those who had received cocaine with those who had not. He noted that animals who had been treated with cocaine lost much more weight than those who had not. These observations are confirmed by modern science, which tells us that cocaine stimulates the production of adrenalin which in turn enhances body metabolism. Freud could have suspected as much since the drug increases the pulse and the body temperature. To Claude Bernard's experiments he responds with the anecdote about the siege of the city of La Paz in 1775,[15] when only those who had taken cocaine survived the famine! He also reminds us that "the nervous system exerts an influence on the feeding of tissues and that psychic factors can cause a healthy man to lose weight. Therefore the sparing effect of cocaine on food consumption and utilization cannot be denied and by stimulating the nervous centers, the drug will affect favorably the feeding of the body." The action of cocaine on metabolism could work, according to Freud, in mysterious ways and through unexplained and unexplainable mechanisms on the nervous centers. Freud is therefore attributing magical powers to the stimulating and euphorizing effects of his miracle drug.

Other experiments conducted in German laboratories were inconclusive, and Freud faults them for the poor quality of the cocaine preparations used. But he is very impressed with a pamphlet on "The Medical Virtues of Cocaine" by an Italian neurologist, Paolo Montegazza,[16] who, according to Freud, "writes so many accurate remarks" that he is "tempted to accept all his observations," even those which he did not "have the opportunity to verify."

Freud does not attach much importance to animal experiments. "Animals of different species," he tells us, "do not have the same sensitivity regarding substances foreign to their organisms. Therefore one shouldn't expect cocaine to affect similarly man and animal." This generalization should be qualified because, although the toxicity of drugs, including cocaine, on different animal species is not identical, it alters certain vital functions in similar ways. Karl Schroff,[17] professor of pharmacology at the School of Medicine of Vienna, and one of Freud's teachers, administered cocaine to rabbits and observed a quickening of the pulse and an increase in blood pressure and in respiratory frequency. With doses of one hundred milligrams per kilo of rabbit weight, convulsions occurred, followed by cardiac and respiratory arrest. Professor Vassili Von Anrep[18] of the University of St. Petersburg made similar observations on dogs.

These pioneer scientists also showed that when its spinal chord is severed near the base of the brain, the animal will not display convulsions or high blood pressure, observations indicating that the drug works through the brain. Freud adds that Schroff "refers to cocaine as a narcotic" (a dependency–producing substance) and "classifies it in the same category as cannabis and opium, whereas all other researchers classify cocaine with caffeine as a stimulant." And yet the leading pharmacologists of his time, such as Lewin and Von Anrep, agree with Schroff that cocaine should be classified among the addictive drugs.

Freud prefers to emphasize the "action of cocaine on healthy [human] individuals," taking himself as an example. "This action, he says, "is similar to chewing coca leaves as described by Mantegazza."

He recalls his first experience, when he swallowed fifty milligrams of cocaine diluted in a little water.

> A viscous solution with, at first, a bitter taste followed by a succession of pleasant flavors. A few minutes later, a sudden playfulness appears, along with a lightheadedness punctuated by light and pleasing belches. This state of euphoria, typical of cocaine, lasts for quite a while, and differs little from a normal, healthy person's euphoric mood. Absent is the drunkenness induced by alcohol.

He also notes dryness of the mouth, but makes no reference to a quickening of the pulse as mentioned by Mantegazza and others.

The most important thing to Freud are cocaine's beneficial effects on mood: he has first a feeling of self-control and
euphoria.

> It seems easier to be in control of oneself, to be stronger, to
> work harder and, while working, to avoid the excitement, the
> surge of mental power caused by tea, alcohol or coffee. Every-
> thing feels normal. It becomes even hard to believe that a
> substance is at work on the mind.

The second remarkable property of coca, its incredible
stimulating action, appears next. "An extended muscular or
mental task can be performed without fatigue: The need to
sleep and to eat seems to have disappeared." As soon as the
effect of coca weakens, one drifts into sleep. "A dozen times, I
have noted on myself how cocaine protects against hunger,
sleep and fatigue and how it maintains the vigilance necessary
to intellectual activity."

Freud never tested on himself the beneficial effect of
cocaine on physical work. He believed there were enough
flawless reports to bear out this effect: witness the case of his
colleague who, after working uninterruptedly for twelve hours,
consumed fifty milligrams of cocaine and felt as if he had
finished a hearty meal; and the story about the seventy-
eight–year–old Englishman who, after chewing eight grams of
coca leaves, walked fifteen miles without feeling hungry,
thirsty or tired.

Freud never consumed large doses of cocaine and merely
quoted Mantegazza,[19] who reports that "after the ingestion of
strong doses of cocaine, his pulse rate was quickened notice-
ably, and his body temperature rose moderately." He subsequently "fell into an euphoric drowsiness, his speech was gar-
bled, and his writing hesitant." Finally he had "bright and
colorful hallucinations, frightening at first but soon to be replaced by a lasting happiness. This cocaine-induced state of
intoxication was not followed by depression or physical discomfort." Freud closes this first section of *Uber Coca* with two
reassuring anecdotes: "Mantegazza never became unconscious
even after consuming sixteen grams of coca leaves. A pharmacist who attempted to poison himself by taking one gram and a
half of cocaine merely developed gastroenteritis and suffered
no mental ill-effects."

From observations on himself and a study of the medical
literature, Freud draws two conclusions.

First, cocaine is not likely to cause physical ill-effects, even when consumed over extended periods in "moderate" doses. Second, the use of cocaine, be it once or on a regular basis, never creates a need for a larger dose; on the contrary, in the long run, a certain repulsion for the substance is likely to appear.

These conclusions are based on unverifiable anecdotes and on personal experiences following the ingestion of doses of cocaine twenty to a hundred times smaller than those self-administered by cocaine addicts. But Freud disregards experimental and clinical reports which describe the toxic effects of the drug on brain and vital functions, and he also fails to diagnose his friend Von Fleishl's[20] irreversible addiction to cocaine.

Freud seems to believe that everyone will consume cocaine as he does, in moderate amounts, and for its beneficial and helpful properties as to mood. But he never defines what he means by "moderate doses," either in frequency or in quantity.

When Freud describes the properties of cocaine he never speaks of the brain. He refers only to the "psychic" effects of the drug — creating euphoria, elevating mood, increasing alertness as if its action were exerted directly on the "mind," and not mediated through brain mechanisms; it follows that the rational mind should control cocaine consumption. In this sense, Freud is more influenced by the classical philosophy and religious thinking of the 17th century Descartes[21] than by 19th century scientific rationalism. Descartes believed in the dichotomy between mind and body, motivated by his profound religious conviction that the beautiful laws of nature had a divine origin. This conviction was absent from Freud's discourse, who seems to attribute to "reason" alone a transcendental power, including that of overcoming cocaine craving. Such thinking was going to lead the great psychoanalyst to a major error of judgment.

7

Cocaine as a Cure For Morphine Addiction:
Freud's "Parapraxis"

The second half of *Uber Coca* is devoted to the therapeutic uses of coca which, according to Freud, were still unknown in Europe although "widely appreciated in North America."[1] "The rejection of this medication is ill-deserved," he claims, and he proceeds to tell us why.

The first therapeutic use of cocaine recommended by Freud is as a stimulant "much more powerful and less dangerous than alcohol." He suggests repeated and well-spaced doses of fifty to one hundred milligrams "during strenuous and extended physical effort without food or rest; in the army or on navy maneuvers; during mountain climbing and excursions." The absence of an ensuing state of depression has already been pointed out, he says, and "none of the physical ill-effects induced by morphine are present."

The stimulating effect of cocaine fills a void in the psychiatrist's remedies, being useful "to increase the reduced activity of the nerve centers and to treat many types of psychic depression; hysteria, hypochondria, melancholia, stupor. Some successful cures have been reported."

Coca has long been a proven remedy for digestive troubles, he goes on. "After a heavy meal it decreases ill-temper and weakness due to 'dyspepsia.' I can personally testify that cocaine heals nausea caused by overeating and restores a normal appetite and a feeling of well-being."

An extended use of cocaine is prescribed by Freud in cases of cachexia or extreme loss of weight resulting from various chronic diseases "such as serious cases of anemia, consumption, persistent fevers, syphilis and prolonged recoveries."

When it comes to "consumptive fever" (tuberculosis), cocaine "controls fever and checks perspiration." The use of cocaine is justified because, he repeats, "a body which receives a dose of cocaine, even a minute one, can stretch its vital strength further."

Turning to studies from the United States, Freud quotes the *Detroit Medical Gazette* to suggest a unique use of cocaine: the treatment of morphine addiction. He mentions his own study of a morphine addict successfully treated with coca (probably referring to Von Fleishl,[2] whose name appears in a review of Freud's original article published in the *St. Louis Medical Journal*[3] in 1886). Freud stresses the fact that "the detoxification process does not mean changing the morphine addict into a cocaine addict. The cocaine consumption is temporary and its action is meant to counter the action of morphine." We also learn that in the United States cocaine is used to alleviate or cure chronic alcoholism and to fight mountain sickness and asthma.

"It appears quite normal that coca should possess aphrodisiac properties since coca chewers in the Andes remain sexually active to a very old age."

Finally Freud acclaims the property of cocaine to anesthetize skin and mucous membranes. He quotes the studies of Dr. François-Charles Fauvel,[4] who calls cocaine "the ideal tensor of vocal cords" and uses it to treat infections of the pharynx. From this long and promising list of therapeutic benefits only the last one, the use of cocaine as a local anesthetic, finds a durable application. This application is explored, not by Freud, but, on his suggestion, by one of his Viennese colleagues, the ophthalmologist Karl Koller,[5] who prepares a cocaine solution and with it anesthetizes the eyeballs of laboratory animals as well as his own. This discovery enthrones Koller in the Hall of Fame of Medicine. Less than a year after the publication of *Uber Coca,* Freud's father was operated on for glaucoma under a local cocaine-induced anesthesia, stamping approval on the medical usefulness of the drug.

Uber Coca brought its author swift fame in medical circles, both in Europe and in the United States. A young and brilliant researcher had proposed a miracle drug. Upon his return to Vienna from Paris where he had visited the famed French neurologist Jean Martin Charcot,[6] Freud published a second edition of his article which was out of print.[7] He added an appendix in which he insisted once more on the great diversity of individual reactions and sensitivities to cocaine: "Some patients are very sensitive to small doses whereas others tolerate amounts up to ten times larger." He also mentions his experiments with a dynamometer, an instrument measuring the strength of the hand's muscular contractions, and he reports that one hundred milligrams of cocaine will double the muscular strength of the hand.

He concludes that "the improved muscular performance should not be attributed to the direct action of the drug on the muscle, but to a heightened feeling of well-being which, in turn, strengthens the motor activity." Here again, Freud's pet theory of the dichotomy between psyche and soma (body) is at work. (In fact, cocaine acts on the muscle and the brain through the same mechanism, the release of adrenaline–like substances.) He reiterates the usefulness of cocaine as a therapeutic agent. "Even subcutaneous injections like those used in cases of stubborn sciatica are totally harmless. For humans, the toxic dose is very high and there seems to be no lethal dose."

A few months later, in March, 1885, Freud presented a paper to the Vienna Psychiatric Society.[8] He describes the euphoria induced by fifty to one hundred milligrams of cocaine taken orally in a water solution by patients who are then relieved from fatigue and asthma for several hours. Again he includes a reference to the treatment of morphine addiction with cocaine as practiced in the United States.

"Cocaine," he says,

> decreases the painful symptoms of the withdrawal syndrome and might even dispel the craving for morphine. I had the opportunity to observe the swift recovery of a morphine addict treated with cocaine. Based on my experiences on the effects of cocaine, my advice in cases of detoxification is to administer subcutaneous cocaine injections of thirty to fifty milligrams without fear of increasing the doses. I have even observed that cocaine rapidly dispels dependency symptoms created by higher and higher doses of morphine. It seems to have a specific action on morphine.

However, the benefits attributed by Freud to cocaine in the treatment of morphine addiction are short-lived. His friend Von Fleishl, the first morphine addict to be "cured" with cocaine in Europe, becomes one of the first European cocaine addicts. The unfortunate Von Fleishl resorts to larger and larger doses of cocaine. Less than a year after the beginning of his treatment he injects himself with one gram a day and falls into a state of mental and physical degradation. He becomes paranoid and Freud recalls the "night of horror" in June, 1885, spent at the side of his delirious and hallucinating friend. Von Fleishl was trying to defend himself against monsters and to rid himself of insects gnawing his skin. Other similar cases of addiction are reported that same year, and Freud is accused by Albrecht Erlenmeyer,[9] one of the greatest psychiatrists of his time and the foremost European specialist on morphine addiction, of unleashing a third scourge on humanity, after alcohol and opium.

This is, according to Freud, "the darkest year of his life," when he is under fierce attacks and has to redefine his position on a drug he praised so highly for its healing virtues.

In his last article on the subject, "Desire and Fear of Cocaine" (1887),[10] Freud finally admits that cocaine should not be used to treat morphine addiction because "it creates a considerably more dangerous threat to health than morphine by triggering a rapid mental and physical deterioration." However, he maintains that cocaine creates no dependency per se and maintains that its intrinsic pharmacological features have never harmed anyone.

Cocaine addiction, declares Freud, now only appears in morphine addicts during a cure where cocaine is the healing agent and creates a new addiction.

> All studies of cocaine addiction and the degradation it causes are related to morphine addicts, individuals already in the devil's clutch. Cocaine in itself has never claimed a victim. Addiction to cocaine and the ills it causes are only to be found in patients whose will has been previously weakened by morphine and who feel the need to be stimulated.

Freud describes his own experience with cocaine and his observations on his patients. He claims that the conditions under which he self-administers the drug preclude any "habit-forming" possibility. "On the contrary, more often than I would have liked, I felt a repulsion for the medication, which forced me to adjust the dosage."

Freud admits the occurrence of acute cocaine intoxication in surgery when the drug is used for local anesthesia, even in small quantities: "These are isolated incidents and no life was ever in danger." However, fatalities due to local anesthesia were already being reported in Freud's time.

He attempts to explain the accidents by stressing once more the individual variability in sensitivity to cocaine, known medically as "idiosyncrasy." He attributes this variability to "an instability of the brain capillary innervation" which varies from person to person and, within the same individual, fluctuates according to time and circumstances. Because an advance determination of the degree of individual sensitivity to cocaine is impossible, Freud recommends "that treatment by subcutaneous cocaine injections of nervous and internal disease be discontinued forthwith." After admitting his past errors, Freud still seeks to have the last word by quoting the studies of the American surgeon general Dr. William Hammond[11] who endorses the use of cocaine in numerous cases and claims cocaine addiction does not exist.

"Hammond," Freud tells us, "self-injected the drug several times subcutaneously and described the light toxic effects that resulted." Actually, Freud did not know that Hammond nearly died of heart and lung failure after a 540–milligram self-injection which promptly rendered him unconscious. In the 1887 paper[12] reporting his near-fatal experience with cocaine Hammond also mentions a young American physician addicted solely to cocaine and who presented the same symptoms as von Fleischl. So Freud feels free to conclude: "There is not one proven case of cocaine addiction, except among morphine addicts who lack the will to interrupt their use of the medication." Of course he was not aware that the famous American surgeon William Halstead[13] of Johns Hopkins University had become severely addicted to cocaine in 1884.

Freud's failure to acknowledge the addictive property of cocaine may be related to his inability to recognize the powerful intrinsic capacity of the drug to impair brain function. Such an oversight leads him to claim that cocaine may be prescribed without ill effects for its euphoric and stimulatory properties on the mind. A similar error of judgment is found among many of his disciples today.

By clinging, against all evidence, to the notion that only morphine addicts can become cocaine addicts, Freud also reinforces the theory that drug addiction is linked primarily to a specific predisposition found in certain individuals, under certain circumstances.[14] Although this psychosocial theory was already questioned one hundred years ago by pharmacologists who were Freud's contemporaries, many psychiatrists to this day fall back on it to explain drug dependency.

After the stir provoked by his paper on cocaine, Freud's enthusiasm for the drug waned and he even declared he had developed a repulsion for a substance that brought him so much grief!

He hoped to reach fame and fortune by revealing the beneficial uses of coca. Instead, he felt guilty because of his friend Von Fleishl's degradation and found himself discredited in the eyes of his peers for having endorsed cocaine treatment for morphine addiction and psychiatric disease.

Although he wrote that there was no lethal dose for cocaine, in 1891, seven years after the publication of the celebrated *Uber Coca,* at least four hundred cases of serious cocaine intoxication, thirteen of them fatal, were reported in the European medical literature.[15]

Freud lost interest in cocaine research and seldom referred to it again in the course of his illustrious career, as if he wanted to bury in the back of his mind a most distasteful episode of his life. He even omits in his successive bibliographies any mention of his 1885 paper before the Vienna Society of Psychiatry, in which he had recommended "without reservation the treatment of morphine addiction with subcutaneous cocaine injections which may be increased in dosage as needed." Neither does he mention his 1887 study, *Fear and Desire of Cocaine.* Freud's biographer has identified these bibliographic omissions as a case of "parapraxis," or involuntary memory lapse due to the subconscious.[16]

Until 1895 Freud remained interested in cocaine and prescribed it to others and to himself in the form of nasal applications for sinusitis. Once he became a full professor, caught up in the treatment of his affluent Viennese clientele, he gradually drifted away from experimental medicine to concentrate on research in the "psychic" areas of hypnotism and in the interpretation of dreams. In 1916, in a letter to his student Ferenzci, he wrote about one of his patients, a cocaine user suffering from hallucinations, and remarked that drug addicts are poor subjects for psychoanalysis "because of their propensity to cling to the security of their drugs."[17]

Psychoanalysis, according to Freud, is counterindicated for the treatment of cocaine addicts whose behavior, modified by the drug, is no longer merely "neurotic." This observation has been forgotten by present–day disciples such as one French psychiatrist who claims that drug addiction is caused by "the broken mirror" syndrome, a metaphor referring to the emotional trauma suffered by the addict in his early relation with his mother.[18]

More recently, some authors have speculated on the possible direct psychopharmacological effects of cocaine on Freud's mental processes, and on the subsequent elaboration of his psychoanalytical theory.[19] The German psychiatrist Jurgen Von Scheidt suggests that it was in 1885–86 when Freud was visiting Charcot in Paris, and consuming cocaine regularly, that he shifted his interest from neuropathology and neurology to psychiatry. Cocaine use, which Freud refers to as a substitute for sex, might have loosened his inhibitions, changed his ego function, and "released sexual and aggressive drives producing a mild regression that privileged the inner world of dreams and fantasy."[20] According to Von Scheidt, Freud's use of cocaine might even have triggered one of his important dreams, "Irma's injection," and explain his subsequent psychoanalytical interpretation.[21] According to this interpretation, cocaine would have helped to reveal to Freud his psychoanalytical interpretation of behavior. "As primitive cultures use drugs to bring the believer into contact with divinity, Freud used cocaine to make contact with the realm of the unconscious."[22] For critics of psychoanalytical theory such as Thornton[23] and Eysenck,[24] if cocaine had such an effect on Freud's brain, it was one of the most unfortunate examples of what this drug can do to distort the thinking of a brilliant and creative mind.

However, Freud was convinced that unlike cocaine, opiates are addictive. He would never forget the fate of Von Fleishl. According to Freud, his friend would not have become a victim of cocaine had he not been first addicted to morphine. As Freud's biographer Ernest Jones reminds us: "Like any good physician, Freud was opposed to the prescription of habit-forming drugs. Suffering from a cancer of the mouth caused by his tobacco addiction, he preferred aspirin to opiates." In *Civilization and its Discontents,* Freud (1930) went so far as to declare: "Certain substances foreign to the body produce immediate pleasant sensations but, at the same time, modify our sensitivity to the extent that unpleasant sensations

escape us. Such is the dangerous and harmful feature of narcotics." Freud must have been referring to heroin, since he
never retracted his original position that cocaine was not
"habit-forming."

He went on ignoring the studies of his two senior colleagues, Albrecht Erlenmeyer and Ludwig Lewin, who shortly
after the publication of *Uber Coca* denounced independently the
medical use of cocaine on the basis of its damaging effects and
profoundly addicting power.

In the late 1980's we have begun to hear a call from some
American intellectuals and even some politicians for the legalization of cocaine. It is therefore appropriate today to review
the observations of Erlenmeyer and Lewin, a century after they
were first published.

8

Erlenmeyer and Lewin's Indictments of Cocaine: "God is a Substance"

Professor Albrecht Erlenmeyer, when he had already reached the top of a prestigious career,[1] deserves the credit for having most promptly and emphatically called to the attention of physicians the major dangers of cocaine which had been indiscriminately prescribed as a wonder drug. Erlenmeyer belonged to a lineage of physicians and scientists famed throughout the 19th and early 20th centuries. One of the most prominent psychiatrists of his era, he was the director of several mental hospitals, wrote numerous treatises emphasizing the organic origin of mental illness, and specialized in the treatment of dependency on opiates, which was at that time mostly medically induced.

He first rebuts Freud's advocacy of the treatment of morphine addiction with cocaine in a paper published in 1885,[2] one year after the publication of *Uber Coca*. This article is followed by a full chapter on cocaine in the third edition of his classic monograph, "Morphine Addiction and its Treatment."[3] "The use of cocaine to treat morphine addiction," writes Erlenmeyer,

> has been publicly trumpeted and praised as a veritable salvation. It was simply a question of propaganda expounded by individuals without any truly scientific experience. They ended up with the sorry and frightening results that use turned into abuse. The genies that they summoned up to help them turned into furies bearing misfortune and disaster.

Erlenmeyer studied cocaine addicts in his clinic and also administered a total of two hundred and thirty-six injections of cocaine to eight morphine addicts and to a number of non-addicted psychiatric patients who were confined in his clinic. As a result of his detailed observations, he concluded that far from being an antidote to morphine addiction, cocaine is an even more damaging drug than the opiate. Erlenmeyer reports the increase in heart rate induced by cocaine, *which* he says, *is also capable of producing serious cardiac disturbances.* He fails to observe any of the favorable effects claimed by Freud, and notes instead mental deterioration, loss of memory, or even paranoid psychosis. Erlenmeyer believed that the proponents of cocaine therapy for morphine addiction mistook the resulting cocaine psychosis for opiate withdrawal symptoms. He was the first to describe apathy, depression, and anxiety as the withdrawal symptoms resulting from discontinuing cocaine. Therefore, writes Erlenmeyer, "one should absolutely not treat morphine addiction with cocaine," and he gives a gloomy prognosis of cocaine dependency, which he believed to be worse than that caused by morphine.

"The picture I have described," concludes Erlenmeyer, is dismal, yet I do not think it somber enough. One who has witnessed the rapid and devastating physical, mental and moral breakdown of a cocaine addict must be most pessimistic concerning the effects of the drug." He even recommends "a total ban on its use, by the competent authorities; oral and subcutaneous administration of cocaine should be forbidden by law; its medical use should be limited to surface anesthesia of the eye and mucosa."

Erlenmeyer's condemnation of cocaine as a general remedy is echoed independently by the best known pharmacologist of his time, Ludwig Lewin.[4] When *Uber Coca* appeared, Lewin was on the pharmacology faculty at the University of Berlin, his alma mater. His first published article, in 1874, reviews chronic morphine addiction and the addict's compulsive behavior with its twin drive: to repeat the original high and to escape the withdrawal symptoms. In 1880 Lewin decided to devote his life to research on the harmful side effects of drugs, thus becoming the first medical toxicologist. In 1881, his first volume, "Secondary Effects of Medications," was published and became a classic work, translated into several languages.[5]

A year after the publication of *Uber Coca,* Lewin responded with an article warning his colleagues against the use of cocaine as a treatment for morphine addiction. "The only result would be a twin passion for the two drugs."[6]

In the following years, and until his death in 1929, Lewin wrote twelve books and nearly two hundred articles, among them a manual on toxicology[7] which went through many printings. Early in his career, Lewin was fascinated by mind-altering and habit-forming substances. He studied two stimulants, betel and kava, which are found in India and Polynesia. He is the first to have described the hallucinogenic effects of the Mexican cactus peyote, which he attributed to mescaline, and of kava kava, which he observed first-hand in Oceania.

He collected most of his research on drugs in his book *Phantastica*[8] which was first published in 1924 and remains a classic in its field. The chapter devoted to cocaine capsulizes forty years of clinical work based on historical and scientific facts. His descriptions and conclusions are as relevant and valid nowadays as they were at the beginning of the century, and deserve to be extensively quoted.

In the introduction, Lewin draws a clear distinction between the legends surrounding coca use in Peru and the historical facts compatible with contemporaneous scientific and medical data. We learn that Indians have been growing and using coca since the fifth century B.C., more than a thousand years before the arrival of the Incas. Conferring a divine origin on the plant was a ploy by the Incas to "reserve it for themselves and turn it into a sacred emblem of power." But gradually the use of the plant spread to the common people, "not for the performance of religious rituals which help humans to rise above themselves and ascend to the superterrestrial but for a more practical reason: the plant's action on the body." Again and again in *Phantastica,* Lewin emphasizes the fact that in primitive societies mind-altering substances are always consumed during religious rites under the supervision of a shaman, or sorcerer, who controls their use.

"The taboo on coca use outside of religious ceremonies, already weakened under the Incas, was permanently wiped out after the Spanish Conquest," observes Lewin. "Since then, little has changed: the quest for euphoria remains the prime goal of the coca user in Andean country. The same quest moves all would-be users throughout the world."

After the conquest of Peru by Francisco Pizarro,[9] in 1554, the new masters of the land encouraged the consumption of coca leaves, which became a currency in which to pay the native workers in the mines and plantations. The harmful consequences to the Indian population did not escape the attention of the religious authorities of the day. In 1567, the Second Religious Council of Lima decreed the use of coca leaves to be "useless, dangerous, [and] a tool of the devil." The Council said that coca "fosters superstitious beliefs and practices among the Indians."[10]

A few years later the viceroy Francisco de Toledo[11] prohibited the practice of using natives in forced labor and paying them with coca leaves because

> this plant is nothing but an invention of the devil. It only appears to give strength by some demonic power. It lacks beneficial virtues and furthermore destroys the lives of many Indians who, at best, leave the plantations in wretched health. For these reasons, in no case and under no circumstances, should they be forced into such work. On the contrary, their health must be protected and their lives preserved.

But the economic interests of the ruling class overrode the political and humanitarian wisdom of the viceroy. The cultivation and sale of coca became a state monopoly which, de facto, legalized the use of coca leaves among the Indians of South America. "It must be noted," warns Lewin, "that since the use of cocaine as a local anesthetic at the end of the nineteenth century, the number of coca tree plantations in South America as well as in Java and Sri Lanka have greatly increased."

The use of coca was ingrained in the life of the Indians, who measured time in terms of the duration of the effects of the drug on the body. Lewin tells us that, for instance, a "cocada" corresponds to forty minutes and represents a couple of miles, the distance a man covers while chewing one mouthful of coca leaves.

Drawing from the same bibliographical sources, Freud and Lewin reach opposite conclusions: Lewin saw cocaine as producing harmful effects on the Indians' mental and physical health, while Freud believed that coca was a most useful ingredient in the life of these same people. Although both men were knowledgeable in the fields of history and anthropology, their interpretation of identical texts differs sharply. Their analyses are fundamentally dissimilar: empirical in Lewin; subjective in Freud, for whom a quasi-mystical speculation on the magic properties of coca prevails over a factual and scientific approach. Interestingly, Lewin was a religious man, a devout practicing Jew,[12] while Freud, also a Jew, openly professed his agnosticism.[13]

Having concluded his historical survey, Lewin examined the effects of the habitual use of coca and cocaine. He distinguished between the ill-effects due to chewing of coca leaves and those resulting from habitual use of cocaine, a "difference of the same order as the one between the effects of morphine and opium."

"However," he adds,

> the use of cocaine and coca leaves presents similar symptoms that may lead to the terminal phase of the cocaine disease. Coca becomes, for the coca chewer, the source of his greatest joys. Under its influence he forgets the daily hardships of reality. He lives in his imagination the pleasures refused to him by his wretched condition.

Lewin admits that chewing coca leaves seems to increase endurance and appease hunger, but he cautions that these deceptive results, in the long run, exhaust the body and undermine health. "Our knowledge of the effects of coca," Lewin explains,

> was at that stage, in 1885, when the essential element of coca, cocaine, was put to medical use. It was then that a physician set forth the sinister idea that cocaine could cure morphine addiction. I promptly objected and predicted that the sole result would be the simultaneous use of the two substances, or what I called the "twin passion." Which is exactly what occurred. And worse still! The initial small doses soon become gradually larger and larger until enormous quantities, one to four and even eight grams, are consumed.

During the following years Freud lost interest in cocaine and cocaine addicts, while Lewin pursued his clinical and experimental work on the addiction, which spread to English and German élites.

> As early as 1901 there are cocaine addicts among men, women, physicians, politicians and writers. After World War I the situation worsens while morphine addiction shows no signs of abating. In large German towns, cocaine addicts can be found in many professions. In bars, restaurants, even on the street, cocaine is illegally sold, mostly in stolen or adulterated forms which reach astronomical prices. In Berlin as reported by his colleagues Joel and Frankel, the police, have discovered one of those cocaine "dens." About a hundred habitues, men and women of all walks of life, including intellectuals and actors, gather together to lose their identity in long sleepy hours.

These people give up everything they own, even their clothing, to reach "the exquisite narcolepsy they so passionately crave." Lewin's moral principles did not permit him to refrain from deploring the degradation of these individuals whose abject state he called "lower than that of animals."

In the third section of his paper Lewin paints a broad picture of cocaine addiction based on observations of hundreds of patients made over more than forty years. Although the biochemical alterations caused to the nerve cells by cocaine were yet to be discovered, Lewin insists on "the intrinsic effect of that drug on the brain." This physiological interpretation by a pharmacologist sharply differs from that of Freud who resorted to vague terms in describing the effects of cocaine on an individual's mood and mind: "infatuation, lightheadedness, euphoria, general feeling of well-being." The psychoanalyst speaks as if the drug acted directly on the "mood and psychic state" without altering the physical condition of the brain.

In clinical terms, according to Lewin, the main symptoms of drug addiction are: a dependency on the substance (specifically, the alkaloid), a gradual increase in dosage, a need to repeat the experience for the pleasing sensations it awakens, and, finally, the collapse into physical and mental misery. The clinical observations are backed by experimental data:

> Unlike what occurs with morphine, animals do not become accustomed to cocaine: repeated doses of this alkaloid induce toxic reactions in the animal: it is possible to conclude that cocaine is more harmful than morphine. Its action on the brain is more brutal. . . . Thus a single injection in the gum or under the skin can provoke serious functional ill-effects on the brain: mental confusion, sensory delusions. Extended usage brings about the gradual development of serious disorders visible in the persistent coca chewers of South America. They become listless, hallucinate and are possessed by their passion for the toxic substance which controls their lives.

To Lewin cocaine is a poison in whatever form it takes and however it is consumed.

> If the use of coca leaves and of cocaine present similar symptoms, cocaine intake has far-reaching consequences, regardless of the way it enters the body. The most common form of ingestion is sniffing. But the drug can be injected subcutaneously, drunk in the form of coca leaf wine or cocainated wine, smoked in cigars, eaten as a powder, spread on the gums or on the oral or genital mucosa.

The harmful effects of cocaine on the brain functions become more and more evident as the irrepressible addiction settles in. Will-power weakens, while indecision, the loss of a sense of duty, capriciousness, stubbornness, memory lapses, and verbal prolixity are aggravated: physical and mental instability sets in. A fastidious person becomes careless, a truthful one becomes deceitful, kind people turn mean and the gregarious seek solitude. One of my patients tells me he has "lost his smile."

The emotional sensitivity often preserved in morphine addicts and a source of momentary well-being is totally lacking in the cocaine addict who appears unable to force upon his new personality a mask of good demeanor compatible with morality or acceptable behavior. His inner unbalance becomes so apparent that he can no longer conceal it. Like the morphine addict, the cocaine user remains blind to his fate for a long time. His intellectual perceptions are so perturbed as to obliterate self-evaluation. A slave to his drug, he lives to satisfy his passion, in the anticipation of a moment in which the best of the present and of the future culminate, even though he is aware of being under the powerful influence of his substance. Mental weakness accompanied by psychic irritability, bitterness towards others, faulty judgment, suspiciousness, erroneous assumptions, a warped interpretation of facts, unjustified jealousy . . . lead the subject, now suffering from insomnia, to a state of delusion, while he remains conscious of what is happening to him.

Seriously ill, the individual is subjected to hallucinations affecting his vision, hearing and taste. He ultimately sinks into mental alienation and hallucinatory madness similar to the alcoholic's "delirium tremens." A profound anxiety due to his delusions grips him. An unfortunate man who had sniffed three grams or more of cocaine armed himself against imaginary enemies. Another one, seized by acute maniac madness, threw himself in the water. Still another one broke dishes, furniture and beat up a friend. Abnormal sensations in nerve endings lead the patient to believe that animals are crawling under his skin. To get rid of them he will mutilate himself or, because of false or imaginary assumptions, attack members of his family. A woman wounded herself with needles while trying to kill her "cocaine roaches." A man suffering from cramps in his limbs thought he was being forcibly electrocuted by wires attached to his body. Explosions of furor and convulsions are the terminal stage of the illness. . . . A cocaine and morphine addict who took daily doses of two grams of morphine and eight grams of cocaine, suffered from epileptic seizures with loss of consciousness followed by total amnesia. Should the preceding dose be increased, fever and respiratory troubles can occur with the convulsions.

According to Lewin, cocaine causes "organic changes" in the chronic user:

I have often observed in the addict somatic and organic afflictions, such as paleness, lack of appetite, weight loss, a decrease in kidney secretion, weakened sexual powers paired with increased erotic desires, a quickening of the pulse, heart palpitations, an irregular cardiac rhythm, abnormal visual and color perceptions, speech difficulties such as stuttering. . . . These disorders increase in frequency and intensity as cocaine consumption rises. Cocaine sniffers have specific symptoms: eczema, an inflammation of the nose, an infection of the septum, which sometimes can become perforated, alteration of hearing and olfactive impairment. The addict's face is often convulsed with tics, he stares ahead and shakes with spasms of irrepressible laughter.

"The addict's future is predetermined," Lewin tells us.

The fortunate ones are so confused by their mental illness that they are unaware of their tragic and fatal destiny. Others have some premonition of being on a dead-end road because of the uncontrollable passion which paralyzes their free will. They only differ from morphine addicts in the extreme devastation of their brain functions by cocaine which ravages, more rapidly and more completely than morphine, any rational behavior or social life.

Lewin lists the crimes committed by cocaine addicts who

break the law in frequent and various ways. The illegal traffic of cocaine, its illegal prescription to addicts, its unlawful purchase have meant numerous jail sentences. There are more serious offenses: thefts, embezzlements, false papers, break ins, armed assault crimes committed to secure either cocaine itself or money to buy it. Some criminal acts include murders and immoral or indecent behavior committed under the influence of cocaine.

Here Lewin pleads extenuating circumstances, claiming the culprit is not responsible for his actions since "the crime is committed by an individual who has lost the exercise of his free will." The addict suffers from insanity.

The accused are nearly always found guilty. However it is hard to believe that the patients are entirely responsible for their actions: it is clear that they are moved by a violent inner compulsion, and are unable to coherently respond to their environment. In turn, any reaction from the outside world only increases their mental confusion. Their confused condition must be viewed as a lasting illness of the mind or a passing morbid mental state. In both cases the subject shows the same psychic disposition: a marked propensity, towards words and actions of a megalomaniac nature. One can therefore conclude that he is not acting of his own free will. The nature of his crime is not in keeping with his true personality and his social position at the time he committed the offense.

In spite of these disastrous consequences, the addict craves so intensely the moment when he falls under the power of the drug that nothing else counts for him, not even his whole future. At the same time, the signs of degradation that point to a fatal conclusion are obvious.

The only effective remedy is an immediate detoxification cure during which the subject will experience withdrawal symptoms. To the outside observer these symptoms seem less serious than those associated with morphine. There are fewer groans, fewer laments, the drug is not so desperately craved. However the withdrawal pains occur in the cells of the brain cortex and are intense and varied enough to make the patient dread a stay in a detoxification center.

A careful study of his patients led Lewin to assert that when deprived of their drug they demonstrated withdrawal symptoms. He thus disassociates himself from Freud and those who, following the lead of that eminent psychoanalyst, espoused his stance. Modern science has vindicated Lewin.

Giving up cocaine, indeed, induces a state of anxiety and depression not marked by dramatic outward signs but nonetheless serious because they are the result of biochemical perturbations. Lewin rightly assumed that cocaine deeply alters those neurotransmitters the brain needs for the orderly transmission of its messages.

Lewin says that for effective treatment total abstinence from the drug is imperative. The addict, according to Lewin, moreover, should remain in a clinic for one year at least. He warns about states of extreme mental anguish and hallucinations.

During the period of abstinence, psychotherapy should be part of the treatment. *But, whatever form it takes, not much can be expected from the cure because the psychic scars caused by the pleasant memories that led to the addiction do not heal completely.* A low percentage of cocaine addicts recover totally. The others relapse.

Lewin's pessimism regarding therapy was based on his own numerous studies and those of his colleagues who attempted to treat cocaine addicts. "These unfortunate people lead miserable lives, each hour marked by the imperious need for a new dose and each new dose worsening the deadly struggle that progresses towards its tragic and inevitable conclusion." He does not hesitate to warn his patients, in writing, of the mortal danger that threatens them. One of them answers back: "My first impression when I read your letter was that you had written my death sentence. You seem to consider my case as desperate and to claim I have no chance of recovery." "Unfortunately," writes Lewin, "although this strong-willed man pulled himself together, decreased his cocaine doses, [he] drank a lot of wine, took veronal, [and] his fate unfolded as predicted."

Lewin reached his conclusions on cocaine after listening carefully to his patients and observing them with the sagacity of a seasoned practitioner. He encouraged them to write to him since he believed that the written word is more accurate than the spoken word in describing in depth a feeling or a subjective sensation. "I can claim in all honesty," writes one of his patients, "that if the past five years have been the best of my life, I owe it primarily to cocaine. Nothing can refute this brutal fact." His twelve–page letter ends with these words: "My concept of the world rests on a single statement: God is a substance." This phrase spells out in the bluntest terms, declares Lewin, the "powerful hold of cocaine on the brain."

There lies the gulf between Lewin's medical and experimental method and Freud's uncertain assumptions based on the interpretation of dreams and associative thinking.

In closing, Lewin did not hesitate to pass a moral judgment on the use of cocaine, a position few scientists feel they can take a century later. "These last few years I have observed the dreadful aftermath of cocaine addiction. Those who imagine they are entering the temple of happiness through the gates of pleasure are buying a moment's bliss at the cost of loss of body and soul."

9

Hans Maier and the Great Cocaine Epidemic at the Turn of the Century

In the years following Erlenmeyer's and Lewin's warnings against the indiscriminate medical use of cocaine, numerous physicians in Europe and the United Sates described many additional examples of the addictive power of this new drug. Cases of addiction were all the more frequent because of its unrestricted sale in pure form by pharmacists and its widespread availability in a large variety of patent medicines: cocaine-containing syrup, lozenges, elixirs, suppositories, ointments were sold over the counter or by mail order and were widely advertised as miracle drugs that would cure any ailment, from the common cold, hay fever, allergies, and sinus troubles to tuberculosis and cancer.[1] Cocaine was also recommended as a treatment for alcoholism and morphine addiction. The Parke Davis Company sold coca leaf cigarettes and cigars and alcohol mixtures of coca ("Coca Cordial"), as well as cocaine-containing tablets, hypodermic injections, and sprays.[2]

The two most famous cocaine-containing products were Mariani Wine in France and Coca-Cola in the United States.[3] Mariani wine was the creation of a young Corsican chemist, Angelo Mariani, who was so impressed by the euphorizing properties of cocaine that in 1864 he decided to make it commercially available in its most palatable form. He macerated coca leaves (thirty grams to a liter, we are told) in sweetened Bordeaux wine. The exact formula of the cordial, which "fortifies and refreshes body and mind, restores health and vitality," was never divulged by its inventor. He took to his grave the secret of the elixir which "protects against malaria, influenza and anemia."

Mariani Wine must have been a popular tonic beverage, since for fifty years in Europe and in the United States its sales kept climbing, backed by a clever publicity scheme that widely reprinted and disseminated the raving letters of the era's great figures. In response to free samples, illustrious families endorsed the wine with rhapsodies of praise. For example, the popular and successful author Anatole France declared "Mariani Wine spreads a subtle fire in the body," only to be outdone by Emile Zola, who referred to this "life-giving elixir." Jules Verne believed that the beverage "can extend a human life a hundred times," and the aviator Louis Blériot admitted he took a bottle with him on his first solo flight across the Channel. Mariani received official approval from the highest religious authorities. Both Pope Pius X and Leo XIII conferred upon him the title of "Benefactor of Humanity."

Crowned heads of Europe, from Spain and Sweden to Imperial Russia, joined President McKinley in hailing the virtues of Mariani Wine. The long list of renowned consumers drew from the ranks of writers such as H. G. Wells and Edmond Rostand, scientists such as Thomas Edison and Nicolas Flammarion, composers such as Gounod and Massenet, the sculptors Bartholdi, the creator of the Statue of Liberty, and Rodin, and the actress Sarah Bernhardt.

In 1886, twenty years after the launching of Mariani Wine, on the other side of the Atlantic an Atlanta pharmacist, John Pemberton, developed a drink he called Coca-Cola, using a formula which remains secret to this day. This beverage originally contained a coca leaf extract with a fair amount of cocaine, caffeine, and some Cola nut. The syrup was prescribed for "headaches, hysteria, melancholia." Within five years the formula was brought by a promoter, Asa Chandler, who used it to make a carbonated drink marketed by the Coca Cola Company; the drink was soon to become hugely successful across the United States. Its popularity rose throughout the world, even after 1904 when the cocaine was eliminated from the coca leaves which remain an ingredient in "Coke."[4]

For several decades pharmacies, groceries, and general stores were stocked with remedies and concoctions containing extracts of coca leaves or cocaine. The leaves were imported in bulk from Peru, Colombia, and Indonesia, while most of the cocaine hydrochloride in its pure form was produced and conditioned in Germany by the Merck Laboratories which shipped the drug to the rest of the world.

Until 1894, when aspirin was introduced into medicine, cocaine and morphine were the only medications available for the rapid relief of pain or discomfort, the common symptoms of all the mental and physical afflictions of man. These two drugs were routinely prescribed separately or in combination by physicians, who had no other effective medicine to treat ailing patients, regardless of the nature of their disease. The selling of cocaine became an exceedingly lucrative business but less so than today, because as sales increased prices fell, which happens with all pleasurable substances in a free market economy.

As a result of the widespread availability of cocaine preparations at modest prices and its generalized prescription by physicians, consumption soared and thousands of consumers became addicted. The most customary use of the drug was by sniffing the powder or ingestion in the form of one of its numerous preparations.

As predicted by Lewin and Erlenmeyer, many who had started with small doses tended to increase their dosages rapidly. The American and European medical literature abounded in case descriptions of addiction to cocaine among people who, though separated by an ocean, presented identical symptoms. Physicians who had easy access to the drug became addicted in large numbers.

One of them, an American, Dr. Ring,[5] reported his own personal experience in "Cocaine and its Fascination" in *The Medical Record* of 1887. A year earlier an editorial in the *New York Medical Record* stated: "There is no other example of a drug which, so shortly after its introduction, has claimed so many victims. Cocaine is a habit more easily acquired than morphine dependence, and its physical and mental effects are much more disastrous."[6] The writer gives the example of a physician and his daughter who behaved in a maniacal fashion after they had taken enormous subcutaneous doses of cocaine. Today, such a report would be described as an "unverifiable anecdote," but it should be examined within the context of the scores of similar reports which appeared at that time in Europe and the United States. In 1886 Dr. D. R. Brower[7] reported a case of "Insanity from Cocaine" in the *Journal of the American Medical Association*; a year later this report was followed by another paper written by the same author, "The Effects of Cocaine on the Central Nervous System,"[8] which appeared in the *Philadelphia Medical Report*. Many other cases of "cocainism" were reported in American medical journals, and in 1898 Dr. J. D. Crothers published "Cocaine Inebriety," a paper in which he describes the spread of cocaine in America.[9]

In the span of a few years the amount of cocaine imported from Germany had increased seven-fold while the price of the drug had been cut in half.[10] Most cocaine addicts injected the drug; the habit was often complicated by morphine addiction and alcoholism. The acute psychiatric reactions associated with cocaine use were often mistaken for alcoholic psychoses. In 1901 Dr. G. W. Norris[11] reported in the *Philadelphia Medical Journal* that close to one third of the cocaine addicts in the United States were physicians or dentists. Many cases went unreported, like the addiction of Dr. William Halstead,[12] one of the great surgeons of the era and a professor at Johns Hopkins. Dr. Halstead became addicted to cocaine after using it to anesthetize nerve trunks and induce anesthesia in whole limbs. A one-year cruise on a sailboat in the Caribbean Islands weaned Halstead from the cocaine habit, but he adopted morphine instead, which he consumed up until his death. Cocaine addiction afflicted people from all walks of life. Simonton, for instance, noted the increased use of cocaine among the people of Pittsburgh, "especially among the blacks who resorted to sniffing the powder while the wealthy injected the substance under the skin."[13] In Cincinnati the number of cocaine addicts, mostly sniffers, was estimated at ten thousand. Simonton also observed that there was a large individual variation in sensitivity to cocaine and that the detoxification period had to last from six months to a year to diminish the chance of relapse.

In 1900, when the United States population numbered one hundred million, the number of opiate and cocaine users ("narcotics") in the United States was estimated at 240,000 by L. Kolb and A. G. DuMetz of the Public Health Service.[14] This figure did not include alcoholics. According to a 1912 official publication by M. J. Wilbert and M. G. Motter of the United State Treasury Department, cases of fatal poisoning, excluding those due to alcohol, numbered 5,000 in one year and the majority were related to opium or cocaine.[15]

In Europe the cocaine epidemic followed a pattern quite

similar to the one which spread over the United States after 1885. However, the medical reports of the damaging effects of cocaine addiction were much more numerous and better documented. At that time medical science and practice were far more developed in Europe than in the United States, where medicine suffered from limited training requirements, weak licensing laws, and a dearth of good medical schools, as emphasized by the Flexner Report of 1910.[16] From the records published in the European literature between 1885 and 1924, any student of cocaine addiction could become familiar with hundreds of clinical and experimental reports describing the effects of this drug. Most of the studies were summarized in Hans Maier's long monograph, *Der Kokainismus* (*On Cocaine*) which was published in 1926, two years after Lewin's review paper in *Phantastica*.[17] Professor Hans Wolfgang Maier was chief of the psychiatric clinic and chairman of the department of Psychiatry at the University of Zurich where he specialized in the study of alcoholism and drug dependence. His book on cocaine not only includes a thorough discussion of three hundred and twenty five texts and articles describing the effects of the drug, but also reports Maier's own clinical observations of one hundred addicts studied in his clinic. Over two thirds of the papers and books reviewed by Maier were published in German, and written by prominent internists, neurologists, pharmacologists, or psychiatrists who all belonged to the prestigious medical schools of pre-war Germany, Austria, or Switzerland. French and Italian medical scientists produced over eighty papers while British and American contributions were limited to twenty–six articles. All of the clinical reports, buttressed by Maier's personal observations, are strikingly similar in describing the mental and physical damage associated with acute or chronic cocaine intoxication and the unique addictive power of this drug. Credit is given to the French physician Magnan[18] for the first description, in 1889, of the tactile hallucinations of cocaine addicts who imagine that insects ("coke bugs") are crawling under their skin. Other hallucinations produced by cocaine, affecting vision and hearing, together with their differences from alcoholic hallucinations, were described by the prominent French neurologist Guillain,[19] whose own experiment confirmed the toxic effects of the drug on the brain. Scores of cocaine "psychoses" or dementia were reported after 1885 by German,[20] Italian,[21] and French[22] authors in terms which were identical to those used by their American colleagues.

In 1904 Albert Stein,[23] a German physician, described the perforation of the nasal septum or partition of the nose and collapse of the nose (saddle nose) following chronic sniffing of cocaine, which nevertheless became the most frequent mode of administration. Other reports followed from France[24] and Russia,[25] where L. Nathanson and L. Lipskeroff reported seventy-four cases of septal perforations between 1920 and 1924 in Moscow.

According to H. Schnyder,[26] cases of death following the administration of the relatively low dose of one hundred milligrams of cocaine for anesthetic purposes were described in 1887.

In 1890 Dr. Edmund Falke[27] reported 176 cases of therapeutic cocaine intoxication which included ten fatalities. Autopsies of two of the victims, who exhibited convulsions, revealed "congestive lesions of heart, brain and lungs." The author reported one case of a fatality following a dose of 0.4 grams while in other instances doses of 1.5 to 5.0 grams were tolerated without any serious symptoms. This large variability in lethal cocaine dose has been reported by different authors up to 1987.[28]

Examination of the records of the dispensing pharmacists can sometimes document the amounts of cocaine consumed by some of the addicts. In 1909 A. Hautant reported the case of a patient who sniffed 10 grams a day.[29] In 1913 K. Heilbronner reported the results of a coroner's inquest concerning one of his patients who developed cocaine paranoid psychosis.[30] The patient, a woman, had obtained the drug from different pharmacists in vials containing 0.3 grams each. Over ten years she had consumed 8771 vials which amounted to 2.6 kilograms of cocaine. One of the pharmacists involved would send her 40 vials at a time. H. Higier, in 1910, reported the case of a German dentist who daily injected himself with 5 grams of cocaine until he developed paranoid psychosis with fits of destructive violence.[31] These reports indicate that many addicts develop a great deal of tolerance to the drug, as Maier also reports for his own patients.[32]

A significant number of the addicted patients described in these reports were physicians or dentists. Among the thirty-five clinical histories described by Maier, one of the seven women and four of the twenty-eight men were physicians. In 1914, Walter Straub, professor of psychiatry at Freiburg in Brisgau, noted the dangers of cocaine intoxication prevalent in large sectors of the population which "one considered the most ambitious and active."[33]

The experimental studies by Italian investigators E. Bravetta and G. Invernizzi reported in 1923 caught my attention.[34] These investigators administered cocaine to dogs and rabbits for four to thirty weeks. At first the animals gradually became tolerant to the drug; with more prolonged intoxication the sensitivity of the animal increased and the effects of the same dose became more marked. After autopsy the animals presented lesions of the lining of the blood vessels, hemorrhages in the brain, and damaged kidneys, and the cardiac cells were broken into segments. Sixty-three years later in our own laboratory, we would be the first to duplicate these same heart lesions in rats to whom we had administered large doses of cocaine.[35] In man, cardiovascular disturbances related to cocaine intoxication were also reported by Maier and his colleagues: "A large dose of the drug induces increase in heart rate, blood pressure, palpitations, and occasionally attacks of angina pectoris, *which should be attributed to a stimulation of the sympathetic system.*" Convulsions and cardiac arrest were the most frequently described symptoms associated with fatalities caused by cocaine overdose.[36] These cases are, according to Maier, underreported "because of insufficient questioning of the people surrounding the victim" and the inaccuracy of the forensic tests for detecting the drug.[37]

"Such acute intoxications," adds Maier, "can be seen following the therapeutic administration of cocaine. In particularly sensitive individuals, even doses below the maximum therapeutic dose of 30 mg., are sometimes sufficient to provoke severe accidents. Many physicians, particularly otorhinolaryngologists, have found themselves in the terrible situation of seeing a robust individual apparently dying a few minutes after an application of cocaine for a trivial surgical intervention. Fatalities of this type were unfortunately quite frequent in earlier days. Even leaving aside the danger of dependence, the possibility of accidents of this type is sufficient to justify total elimination of cocaine from the medical and therapeutic arsenal and its replacement by an equally effective derivative which is free of this danger, such as psicaine.

Nowadays with the availability of other more effective synthetic derivatives such as procaine, lidocaine, and related substances, the recommendation of Maier is even more justified than when he first made it.

After a thorough analysis of the effects of cocaine on sexual activity, Maier concludes that "the physical manifestations of sexuality are markedly stimulated in women and inhibited in men, while the libido and erotic imagination are stimulated in both."[38] He also believed like his colleagues E. Joel, F. Frankel,[39] H. Piouffle,[40] and N. Marx,[41], that homosexuals have a particular predilection for the drug and that heterosexuals under the influence of cocaine engage in homosexual activity.

Maier, like Lewin, is very reserved concerning the prognosis and treatment of cocaine addiction.[42] The prognosis of life–threatening acute intoxication must be made very cautiously because there is a large individual variation in lethal dose and no specific treatment, he said — a situation which is quite similar to what it still is today. As for the treatment of the chronic case,[43] he believes that only mild ones may be treated as out-patients. For the vast majority, confinement to a closed institution for six to twelve months under firm and rigorous surveillance should be mandatory, and all addictive drugs including alcohol should be withheld. In any case, says Maier,

> cocaine can and should be withdrawn immediately every time a patient request medical help.[44] The physician does not have the right to prescribe cocaine even to the most confirmed addict. The physician who yields to such demands makes a professional mistake for which he should be accountable. The only attitude that the physician must adopt when confronted with chronic cocaine use of any type, is to absolutely forbid the patient to use the drug.

Maier could not even conceive of accepting recreational cocaine use. The prolonged period of rehabilitation required for the treatment of cocaine addiction was also recommended by Lewin and Maier's colleagues, but it does not ensure a permanent cure, which is "no more frequent than those of morphine addiction and perhaps less so."[45] Symptoms of cocaine psychoses disappear quickly after abstinence from the drug but reappear in the same form after each intoxication. In many cases the patients, following a series of treatments, will relapse and die of overdose, suicide, or intercurrent infections facilitated by physical debility.

Maier devotes an entire chapter of his book[46] to the social dangers of cocaine addiction and its legal control. Like his colleagues Victor Heineman,[47] and H. Zangger[48] and many French specialists, he believes that every cocaine addict must be considered as affected by a contagious disease and consequently as a public danger. He believes isolation is the only way of protecting society from the contagion. Such a firm attitude was based on Maier's personal observations which led him to conclude that cocaine users, especially sniffers, much more so than morphine addicts, are proselytes: "The ease and simplicity of sniffing, and the need of the cocaine user to seek the company of others cause an immense wave of cocaine use to spread rapidly through all civilized countries and especially through large urban centers." Cocaine, unlike morphine, "stimulates mental process which become fully concentrated on the surroundings; under the influence of the drug, addicts express profusely all of their fantasies and become very sociable; they reinforce their mutual euphoria and elation, which are enhanced because commonly shared."

Maier claims that, according to his personal experience, a single cocaine user is capable, in the space of several weeks, of recruiting dozens of other individuals. And each new recruit can, in turn, become a new focus of contagion. He gives an example, which he observed himself, of a district in a medium-sized town which, a few years after the first World War, became within three months a center of cocaine addiction. It all started with a couple who owned a tobacco store which became an outlet for cocaine powder. They became addicted themselves and their addiction spread to their neighborhood, involving dozens of industrial workers, shop owners, and middle-class people.

This observation, says Maier, indicates that cocaine spreads "not only among the wealthy who may squander their money indiscriminately" but to all social classes. Maier also describes the addicted consumer who has to become a small dealer in order to satisfy his own habit and who adulterates the cocaine he sells in order to increase his profit.

The small addicted dealer gets his supplies from large-scale dealers who are rarely addicted themselves and belong to well-knit organizations. "The small dealer is usually arrested by the police while the supplier generally escapes." More than sixty years after Maier's observations, the same pattern of cocaine traffic emerged in the inner cities of America. Instead of cocaine hydrochloride, a much more addictive and damaging substance was traded by dealers who sold cocaine base or "crack," which was smoked instead of sniffed.

Maier is also concerned about cocaine-related criminality. He distinguishes three types of crime-related cocaine users.[49] First there are those who resort to cocaine to stimulate their criminal intent and bolster the aggressivity required for a burglary, an armed robbery, or an assault. They are the criminals using cocaine. Second, there are others who are the victims of cocaine dealers, who have been given cocaine in order to make them easy prey: for instance, women who are raped or robbed while under the influence of the drug. And finally, there are cocaine users who have become violent or paranoiac as a result of taking the drug, and who will commit murder or suicide. It is this social concern of Maier which led him to cooperate with the police and even to take part in investigations and to lead a campaign aimed at establishing restrictive laws on cocaine use in Switzerland. He was merely the spokesman for his colleagues and all practicing physicians as well as other professional and civic leaders. On his initiative, the Swiss Psychiatric Association in a special meeting on November 27, 1921, made the following recommendations:[50]

1. Cocaine addicts, who always represent a public danger, shall be officially confined to closed institutions.
2. Illicit traffic or illicit possession shall be subject to severe penalties.
3. Production, importation, or exportation of cocaine shall be subject to rigorous control.

This initiative led the Swiss government to abandon its legendary neutrality and to take part in the international fight against "narcotic substances" by adhering to the Hague Convention of 1912 and the Geneva Convention of 1924.

Maier ends his book on a note of forceful commitment. "In most countries public health authorities, elected representatives, courts of law, and the police are equally eager to fight against this type of addiction, so dangerous from a social point of view." And the author goes on to formulate a series of practical recommendations which most physicians of the time endorsed. "It must be emphasized," says Maier,

that each cocaine addict is a dangerous source of contamination and that numerous traffickers, often addicted themselves, have a vested interest in increasing the size of their clientele by spreading the use of the drug. It is therefore important to adopt administrative and legal measures including permanent confinement of recidivists that will permit the institutional treatment of these patients *even against their will.*

The consequences of illicit traffic, adds Maier, are no less dangerous than those of severe bodily assault. The punishment should consist of long imprisonment and, in the case of guilty medical personnel, of suspension of their license to practice.

Maier is aware that

complete elimination of the illicit traffic will not occur until rigorous and full control of the amounts of cocaine produced or imported into each country from the point of production to the point of use is achieved so as to preclude completely any deviation to the illicit market. To be effective the fight against cocaine addiction, therefore, requires international agreements, since the drug is manufactured in only a few countries, and large-scale smuggling has developed.[51]

In this statement Maier was referring to Germany, Switzerland, Austria, and France where cocaine was then extracted from imported coca leaves by large pharmaceutical firms for medical or apothecary use. If control of European cocaine manufacture could be readily achieved by international agreement, this was not the case elsewhere, as Maier notes with great foresight: "It should be remembered that the extraction of cocaine from coca leaves is a very simple operation which can be undertaken by small factories located in overseas countries and especially conceived for that purpose."[52] Maier is also convinced, like his colleague Walter Shaub, professor of pharmacology at the University of Freiburg in Brisgau, that it should be possible to develop a series of cocaine derivatives which would have the anesthetic properties of cocaine but none of its potential for abuse. Such a discovery would eliminate cocaine from the pharmacopia and thus from the stocks of legitimate drugs, which are the main cocaine source for the population at large.

But there would still be a danger of illicit production of cocaine for non-medical purposes. Therefore, concludes Maier,

We will have to rely on individual methods of prevention. It will be incumbent upon us to protect the youth of our large cities from the temptation of resorting to unhealthy sources of pleasure by training it to acquire healthy recreational habits. This will not be enough. In addition, the medical profession, the authorities, the pharmaceutical industry and the pharmacists, as well as the police and the courts of all countries will have to make a united and concerted effort not only to bring about legislation against the most dangerous drugs among which cocaine unquestionably belongs, but, above all, to ensure its implementation. [53]

The closing sentence of his book expressed the hope of a bygone era:

Although it is common to discuss the horrors of chemical warfare, not enough attention has been paid to the much larger public danger posed by the threatening spread of the non-medical use of strong intoxicants, such as cocaine. It is still possible and probably not too late to eradicate this addiction if it is caught at an early stage of its development. Let us hope that we are so successful in these efforts that cocaine addiction will be of value only to the historian of medicine interested in the study of the mistakes and errors of judgment of our phase of civilization!

It is most unfortunate that Maier's remarkable contribution to the clinical knowledge of cocaine addiction and its complications was ignored by his colleagues even as late as fifty years after it was published and hardly twenty five years after his death. However, his efforts were not totally in vain, since they led to the implementation of restrictive laws against cocaine use and a temporary containment of the epidemic. Indeed, during the early part of this century the leading European and American pharmacologists, physicians, and psychiatrists overwhelmingly supported and even, at times, like Maier, initiated restrictive laws against cocaine.

This medical consensus largely contributed to create and maintain for several decades in the Western world a taboo against the recreational use of cocaine, and supported national and international legislation which repressed its illicit use and traffic.

In this great humanitarian crusade, the United States led the way.

10

Restrictive Laws against Cocaine: From National to International Legislation

Laws aimed at curtailing the use of morphine and cocaine were enacted at the state level in the last decade of the 19th century. The first one was passed in Illinois in 1897.[1] By 1912, a large number of the states of the Union had adopted special measures forbidding the dispensing of cocaine except on prescriptions issued by registered physicians and veterinarians. Public schools of fourteen states included courses on the harmful effects of alcohol, morphine, and cocaine. Some state laws stipulated that cocaine or morphine addiction, as well as alcoholism, was grounds for divorce. In other states physicians and dentists were forbidden to issue cocaine to recognized cocaine addicts. The simple listing, without comment, of all the legislative measures taken in the United States during the last decade of the century to control dangerous or addictive drugs filled a 209-page volume published by M. J. Wilbert and M. G. Motter[2] in 1912 under the title *Digest of Laws and Regulations in Force in the United States Relating to the Possession, Use, Sale and Manufacturing of Poisons and Habit Forming Drugs.* But loopholes in all of these measures permitted the diversion of opium and cocaine to non medical use, because the states had no cohesive policy to prevent the commercial spread of these habit–forming drugs.

If one state had strict laws, like New York, its neighbors like New Jersey had weak ones, a situation which prevented overall uniform control. The power of the federal government was restricted to regulation of interstate commerce and levying taxes, and federal control over narcotic use and the prescription practices of physicians was thought by many to be unconstitutional. Law enforcement and health-related problems were responsibilities of the states. So it took the able leadership of public–spirited statesmen, and the broad support of pharmacists, physicians, and clerics, to muster the national consensus required for the adoption of federal restrictive legislation of addictive drugs within the framework of the Constitution. Many of these reformers belonged to the Progressive movement, and believed that local and state governments should be given federal guidelines to preserve the environment and public health against the encroachments of private interests. The reform movement aimed at restricting to medical purposes the use of addictive drugs, though federal legislation was initiated under the leadership of President Theodore Roosevelt.[3] Roosevelt was assisted in this endeavor by three most able men: Dr. Harvey Washington Wiley, a chemist; Dr. Hamilton Wright, a physician and diplomat; and Episcopal bishop Charles Henry Brent, who provided a moral thrust to the lay reformers. All three men independently and at times concurrently laid the basis of the federal legislation first embodied in the Pure Food and Drug Act of 1906, and which culminated in the Harrison Act of 1914. The first federal provisions that required information as to content and accuracy of claims for proprietary drugs were contained in the Pure Food and Drug Act. Any over-the-counter remedy in interstate commerce containing opiates, cannabis, or cocaine had to specify on the label the content and amount of any of these substances. Before its enactment by Congress in 1906, the Act had been approved by the American Pharmaceutical Association, and its implementation was placed in the Bureau of Chemistry of the Department of Agriculture headed by Dr. Harvey Wiley.[4] Wiley had created this bureau to control the manufacture of food products and beverages so as to eliminate from public consumption any substance dangerous to health. In fact, the Pure Food and Drug Act added addictive drugs to the list of substances presenting a health hazard and which had to be controlled. Supported by the pharmaceutical industry, Wiley implemented the provisions of the new Act with vigor. As a result, in the following years the sale of patent medicine containing opiates or cocaine dropped by one third. But large sales still continued in grocery stores and through mail order houses.

In 1908 Wiley prepared an amendment to the Pure Food and Drug Act which would have eliminated any medicine containing addictive drugs from interstate commerce except under the prescription of a physician.[5] But at that time the United States had become a world power with commitments in the Far East where the control of opiates required much more far-reaching national and international legislation. At this juncture the leading proponent of such legislative measures shifted from the Agriculture Department's Bureau of Chemistry to the State Department[6] and focused on the control of the flourishing opium trade in Southeast Asia. (By contrast cocaine, at that time, was manufactured by a few pharmaceutical firms in Germany and in the United States, and its traffic could be much more readily controlled.) The United States, in order to secure its share of the commercial markets of China, had to help that country overcome its massive consumption of opium largely caused by British mercantilism since the Opium Wars.

Another problem for the United States was to provide the Philippine Islands, which they had wrested from the Spanish at the turn of the century, with the proper measures to control the widespread consumption of opium in the islands.[7] The United States policy in China as well as the Philippines was greatly influenced by the Right Reverend Charles Henry Brent,[8] who was appointed in 1902 as the first Episcopal bishop of the Philippines. Not only did he develop schools and hospitals in the Islands, but he provided a moral conscience for the Philippine Commission that managed the Islands. Held in high esteem by the Philippine governor William Howard Taft and by President Theodore Roosevelt, Bishop Brent also played a major role in formulating the international legislation for opiate control in the Philippines and China.

His philosophy was simple. Drug addiction was a social problem which required a moral approach in order to reach a solution. Cocaine and opium had no value other than as medicines. Unlike alcohol, they had no caloric value, and they were unlikely to be consumed in moderate amounts in a regular fashion because of their addictive potential. There was no justification for their non-medical use, only a risk of becoming addicted. Therefore the recreational use of these substances should be prohibited, their traffic curtailed on a world scale, and a plague eliminated from the surface of the earth. This philosophy might have been based on moral grounds, but Bishop Brent had an open mind, and at the request of Governor Taft, in 1903 he made a fact-finding tour of the Far

Eastern countries (Japan, China, Indochina, Burma, Java). He concluded, "The only effective laws, are those enacted by Japan, and it is somewhat after the Japanese model that we will mold our suggestions."[9] His main recommendation was gradually to prohibit opium consumption in the Philippines except for medical purposes.[10] In 1905 Congress approved the recommendation of Bishop Brent's commission, placing a three–year limit on the transitional period until total prohibition of the drug.

After resolving the opium problem in the Philippines, the United States turned to the opium trade in China, at a time when anti-American sentiment there was rife and only matched by the anti-Chinese xenophobia in the U.S. But it was important to consolidate, by an international treaty, the 1906 British-Chinese agreement, which concurrently abolished import of opium from India and opium cultivation in China. Bishop Brent then wrote to Roosevelt[11] urging an international meeting of the great powers and Japan, to help China with its anti-opium struggle and to consolidate opiate prohibition in the Philippines.

The American reformers and political leaders of the time were convinced that the limitation and control of the sources of production of opium in China and the Far East was essential in order to limit opium entry into the United States. The U.S. in turn was obliged to promulgate its own restrictive national legislation as an example to other countries. Adoption of interdiction measures abroad could also be used to prod Congress and the American public to formulate similar measures at home.

Roosevelt enthusiastically supported Bishop Brent's proposal. It was time to assuage the Chinese resentment against America, and compete with European powers for the Chinese markets.[12] Roosevelt initiated the conference by inviting all of the great European and Asian powers to convene in Shanghai, and appointed a three–man commission to represent the U.S. They were Dr. Hamilton Wright,[13] a physician who had studied tropical diseases in the Far East; Dr. Charles Tenney, a former missionary to China; and Bishop Brent, who served as chairman. The Shanghai Opium Commission met in February of 1909. There was unanimous agreement that drastic measures should be taken by each government to control morphine and other opium derivatives. Such a resolution gave the American representatives to the Commission, Bishop Brent, and especially Dr. Wright, strong arguments to press at home for forceful anti-narcotic legislation. It was a struggle in which, as a state department officer, Hamilton Wright became so deeply involved that he has been called the real father of the anti-narcotic legislation embodied in the Harrison Act. The Act was finally adopted in December of 1914. In the intervening years, Dr. Wright continued his fight on two fronts, domestic as well as international. At home, he was unable to overcome the objections of the pharmaceutical industry and maneuver through Congress a strong anti-drug bill (the Foster Bill),[14] in spite of the strong support given him by the new President, William Howard Taft. But Dr. Wright was able to organize the first Opium Conference, which assembled the representatives of twelve nations.[15] They met in the Hague in December of 1911 to consider ways to regulate international narcotic traffic. The Conference was chaired by Bishop Brent, who symbolized the American moral stewardship.

The resulting treaty restricted narcotics to medical use only and was the basis of legislation to control production of cocaine and opium, their manufacture into pharmaceutical preparations, their distribution within each nation, and their international export. A year later the Convention was signed by all participating powers, and Dr. Wright resumed his efforts to pass suitable domestic legislation. Backed by the adamant reformer Dr. Alexander Wiley, he enlisted Representative Francis Burton Harrison to shepherd the legislation through the House. Two years were required for the passage of this Act, which was finally signed into law by President Woodrow Wilson on December 14, 1914 and gave the United States effective restrictive legislation against the non-medical use of cocaine and opiates. The Harrison Act[16] required the registration of every dealer in "narcotics" with the Bureau of Internal Revenue. All transactions required detailed record keeping, and a physician's prescription was necessary to obtain a registered drug. The purpose of this reform was to prevent the dispensing of addictive drugs to addicts.

This Act was timely. A 1910 health survey found that there were still 250,000 habitual users of opiates and of cocaine in a nation which then numbered less than one hundred million people.[17] Passage of the Harrison Act was a bipartisan achievement. The law was drafted after consultation with the medical profession, pharmacy representatives, and pharamceutical companies. Reform groups provided active support which was based on a national consensus. By 1914, newspaper editors, physicians, pharmacists, judges, and elected representatives believed that cocaine and opium were dangerous substances alien to the American way of life, and that they should be strictly regulated.

These drugs were perceived to be far more damaging than alcohol, and there was a public as well as a congressional distinction between narcotic control and liquor prohibition.[18] This perception was based on the many clinical observations by physicians and laymen alike who had witnessed the rapid and often uncontrollable development of cocaine or morphine addiction after a few weeks of daily exposure to the drugs. Passage of the Act was also a great victory for the reformers. They were convinced that a strong anti-narcotic legislation at home aimed at a drastic curtailment of the demand for non-medical use of addictive drugs was a paramount measure. It was essential for the implementation of steps required to control the supply and trade of "narcotics" in the producing countries.

The Harrison Act had the support of the A.M.A.,[19] American Medical Association, which was led by a small group of physicians who were influenced by the reform movement of the Progressive era. The most vocal physician reformers were Dr. Alexander Lambert,[20] head of the A.M.A. Judicial Council, and Dr. George Simmons,[21] editor of the Journal of the American Medical Association (J.A.M.A). They supported the Pure Food and Drug Act, uniform procedures for medical licensing, and antinarcotic legislation such as the Harrison Act. In later years through fear of federal intervention in the practice of medicine, the A.M.A. was lukewarm in supporting any federal legislation in the health field.[22] Scientists and businessmen also rallied to support strict anti-narcotic legislation, one of them being Dr. William Schieffelin, a chemist who headed the Committee of One Hundred on National Health formed in 1910 and a model of the Progressive era's public-spirited businessmen.[23]

But Dr. Wright, in the course of his protracted fight to secure this new legislation, alienated many of his friends and foes alike. He was not selected to participate in the Third

Opium Conference held at The Hague in 1914, on the eve of the First World War, and was dismissed from the State Department that same year.[24]

One year after the Hague Conference of 1914, and passage of the Harrison Act, restrictive laws passed in Europe and in the United States cleared grocery and pharmacy shelves of all miracle medications laced with opium or cocaine. The market for Mariani wine was wiped out, and its French inventor died a few months before the enforcement of the legislation that banned his elixir of life. These belated measures to protect society from cocaine vindicated Erlenmeyer's and Lewin's medical indictment of the drug, while rebutting Freud's opinion of the beneficial effects of its moderate use.

As could be expected, the strict interpretation of the Harrison Act, which banned the prescription of opiates to opium addicts, was challenged in the courts. The famous *Jin Fuey Moy* Supreme Court decision of 1916 held that such a provision infringed individual rights.[25] Three years later the Court, in an about-face, made it illegal for physicians to prescribe addictive drugs for maintenance treatment of addiction.[26] This 5 to 4 decision was carried with the vote of Justice Oliver Wendell Holmes, a Theodore Roosevelt appointee, and marked the triumph of the reformers. As no cure was more effective than just keeping the addict away from drugs, it appeared to most citizens that society did not have a medical problem to solve, but rather an enforcement problem.

In 1919, A. G. DuMez, an official of the Treasury Department's special committee entrusted with the enforcement of the Harrison Act, declared in a memorandum to the Surgeon General: *"The medical profession has awakened to the fact that addiction to the use of 'narcotics' produced changes in the organism which cannot be controlled by the will power of the individual. Our present methods of treating drug addiction must be considered failures."*[27]

A narcotic division was formed as part of the Prohibition Unit of the Internal Revenue Bureau in 1919 in order to enforce the Harrison Act strictly. All maintenance clinics, numbering about forty throughout the nation and servicing about 5000 addicts, were closed between 1918 and 1925.[28] The general experience of these clinics was that maintenance merely perpetuated addiction and seldom led to a cure.[29]

The medical profession objected to the Harrison Act as an infringement by the federal government on the free exercise of medicine; many physicians resented what they considered interference in their right to prescribe.[30] They grudgingly complied with the federal law, however. The Harrison Act was upheld again by the Supreme Court in 1928,[31] and it became the main deterrent to drug addiction, under the unrelenting pressure of the Narcotic Division of the Prohibition Unit.[32]

After the outlawing of opiate maintenance for addicts, a series of federal laws were enacted between 1922 and 1930 to strengthen narcotics control. The Narcotic Drugs Export and Import Act (1922)[33] permitted only crude narcotics to enter the U.S.; the manufacture of the pure substance was to be performed by the drug companies. Next, Congress under the initiative of Ohio congressman Stephen Porter, who had assumed congressional leadership in the field of narcotics, prohibited opium importation for heroin manufacture (1924).[34]

After the first World War, the United States was foremost among nations in passing the most stringent legislation against cocaine and heroin usage for other than medical or scientific purposes and was therefore in a strong position to sponsor and even charter the international control of the traffic in these illicit drugs. Though the United States was not a member of the League of Nations, it participated in the second Opium Conference held under the auspices of the League in 1924–25.[35] The United States send a blue-ribbon delegation led by Representative Porter and including Bishop Brent and former Surgeon General Rupert Blue. Their goals was to obtain a world-wide halt of heroin manufacturing, similar to the ban voted by the U.S. Congress in 1924. They also believed that a strict control over the growing of poppies and coca bushes was an essential step to limit the manufacture of opium and coca derivatives.[36] The United States delegates and especially Congressman Porter found out that they were ahead of their time: The opium-producing nations, with the exception of China and Egypt, were not in agreement with the American position and obstruction came from India, represented by its British rulers. The conference would not agree to ban the manufacture of heroin, or to lower the level of narcotics permitted in exempt preparations, or to take steps to suppress opium smoking in the Far East. The substitution of *recommendation* for an *obligation* to apply the restrictions of the Convention to dangerous new drugs riled the State Department. However, positive steps were taken: the establishment of a League advisory committee, procedures for the sharing of statistics, and measures to encourage cooperation between national narcotics enforcement administrations were adopted, as well as a resolution to add cannabis to the list of controlled substances which, by international agreement, were to be limited to medical and scientific usage.[37]

But the American delegation was unable to obtain a commitment from Great Britain, India, Persia, and Turkey to restrict opium production or a commitment from Peru, Bolivia, Java, and The Netherlands to curtail coca bush plantations. Therefore Porter walked out of the conference with the American delegation, so convinced was he that the production of raw opium and the growing of the coca bush must be controlled at the source before any other aspect of narcotics traffic could be effectively addressed. Without such basic restrictions, Porter claimed, international regulation of drug manufacturing and domestic laws such as the U.S. Harrison Act were in jeopardy.

The epidemic of cocaine addiction besetting America today has proved that Porter was right. His far-reaching goal of eradicating addictive drugs at their source, premature for his time, remains the only long-term solution, and still might be reached before the end of the century through the concentrated efforts of the United Nations.

It was in the area of narcotic control that the United States, under the guidance of Presidents Theodore Roosevelt, William Howard Taft, and Woodrow Wilson, exercised global leadership, for the first time in its history, during the early part of the 20th century. It was leadership aimed at the betterment and protection of the common man and at the strengthening of the democratic process by defending basic human values, a leadership which found its full expression during and after the Second World War, when America became the leader of the free world, supporting freedom against tyranny with all of its power.

The exemplary commitment of the United States to control the traffic in cocaine and opiates was welcomed by many European statesmen during and after the First World War. Addiction to cocaine was more prevalent in Europe than the use of opiates and the unsurpassed addictive power of cocaine was recognized by most European physicians. In 1916 France passed a special law against cocaine traffic and its nonmedical use which was widespread in Paris, even among school children, according to Giroux.[38] Penalties, including banishment and long prison sentences, were voted by the French Parliament in 1923, in an attempt to curtail a burgeoning illicit trade;[39] similar measures were taken in Germany, the nations of central Europe, and Switzerland,[40] and all of these interdiction measures proved most effective.

At the next Geneva Conference on the limitation of the manufacture of narcotic drugs held under the aegis of the League of Nations in 1930, which was attended by fifty-seven countries, the European nations welcomed the return of the United States delegation.[41] The resolutions arrived at during this convention represented a marked improvement over previous international agreements. Heroin could not be exported upon the mere request of an importing nation. Careful recording and reporting of all raw materials would be required. A separate narcotic agency in each government was requested. But action on the United States' main goal of controlling the production of opium and coca at the source was postponed again to a future time. The last international meeting held before the war and attended by the United States was called by the League of Nations in 1936 for the suppression of the illicit traffic in dangerous drugs. Its aim was to improve detection of illicit traffic and increase the penalties imposed on those who violated narcotics laws.

All of the national and international legislation enacted between the two great wars to curb the traffic of addictive drugs and their recreational use met with a good measure of success in the United States and around the world. Between 1920 and 1940, cocaine addiction was observed only in a few marginal sectors of high society. The rejection by a broad social consensus of a behavior linked to delinquency and deviancy was approved by the media to the extent that "recreational" drug use was not socially acceptable.

In 1930, on the initiative of Congressman Porter, the United States Congress established a separate government agency, the Federal Bureau of Narcotics (FBN) to enforce the Harrison Act and represent the United States at foreign conferences.[42] Harry Anslinger, a former diplomat, became the first Commissioner of Narcotics, and directed the Federal Bureau of Narcotics in a highly efficient fashion until his retirement in 1962.

When Anslinger took office the problem of opiate and of heroin addiction appeared to be receding under the thrust of the Narcotic Division of the Prohibition unit. The "narcs," as they were called, led by Levi Nutt,[43] strictly implemented the Harrison Act even against physicians who prescribed opiates for maintenance. High fines and mandatory sentences were imposed for a first offense. As a result of this policy it was estimated that the number of addicts had fallen to around 100,000 in 1930.[44] Convicted narcotic law violators were sent to Federal prisons where they numbered up to nearly one third of the incarcerated population, and in April of 1928 they were 2300 out of 7600 federal convicts.[45]

Porter introduced legislation that same year to create special detention quarters, dubbed federal narcotic farms, for convicted addicts.[46] He also surmised that these institutions might provide some type of treatment for addicts. Two such farms, operated by the Public Health Service, were created, one in Lexington, Kentucky, the other in Fort Worth, Texas. They were the first attempt at compulsory "treatment" or rehabilitation of addicts. The recorded cure rate was modest, no better or worse than any form of treatment available at that time. There was disaffection with these farms in the 1960s when the medical model of dealing with drug addiction replaced the penal model. At best the narcotic farms were the first attempt to rehabilitate addicts as a group, with a drug-free life as a therapeutic goal. This model was adopted successfully by the Japanese in the 1950s and subsequently by the therapeutic communities around the world.

During the 1930s, the combined effect of the Great Depression and continued enactment by the Federal Bureau of Narcotics of a policy of imposing fines and mandatory jail sentences for first offenders resulted in a further decrease in the number of addicts. This number, according to Anslinger, had reached 60,000 in 1936, which corresponded to a per capita ratio in the population of 1 in 3000, down from 1 in 500 before the Harrison Act.[47] This low rate of addiction was achieved while the budget of the Bureau of Narcotics stabilized for the entire decade at a modest figure, averaging between $1.1 to $1.5 million annually.[48] The number of enforcement agents even declined, never exceeding 300.[49]

Cocaine addiction was on the wane during that whole period. New synthetic local anesthetics such as novacaine became available in 1932. Free from the addictive properties of cocaine, they were widely adopted by the medical and dental professions, and the risk posed by cocaine of medically induced addiction was thus eliminated.

Anslinger was able to concentrate his efforts on measures aimed at controlling, in the United States, the non–medical use of cannabis (marijuana), a drug which with heroin and cocaine had been targeted for restrictive legislation at the Second Opium Conference of 1925.[50] The Marijuana Tax Act sponsored by the Federal Bureau of Narcotics was passed by Congress in 1937; the Act banned the cultivation, possession, and distribution of hemp plants, except for the mature stalk, which was used in the manufacture of twine and cordage. With the passage of the Marijuana Tax Act, the United States was simply following the recommendation of the 1925 International Opium Conference that placed cannabis in the same category as the opiates and cocaine. Anslinger and the Federal Bureau of Narcotics were also responding to a grassroots cultural movement in the United States which, at that time, was opposed to the use of all mind-altering drugs.[51]

According to the FBN, in the period from 1925 to 1939 the number of opiate addicts in the U.S. was reduced from 250,000 habitual users to approximately 50,000, which represents an 80% drop, and in reference to the overall American population a 90% decline.[52]

In Europe the number of cocaine and opiate addicts also declined as a result of a generally disapproving social climate as well as law enforcement efforts directed against drug traffic. The use of cannabis was practically unknown.

Egypt, which had been in the grip of a widespread epidemic of cocaine and intravenous heroin addiction in the 1920s, was able to stamp it out, thanks to the efforts of Thomas Russell, the British narcotics commissioner.[53] He accomplished this remarkable task with the support of the Egyptian government and of the League of Nations, and was able to dry up the supplies of cocaine as well as of heroin by enforcing strict methods of interdiction directed towards suppliers and consumers alike.

The use of addictive drugs in the United States and the western world declined in the era between the two world wars, as a cultural and medical consensus supported a repressive policy, a consensus which was still stronger in continental

Europe than in the United States or England. And so on the eve of the Second World War the United States and its traditional allies had, to a great extent, won a long, hard fight against "recreational use" of opiates, cocaine, and cannabis. In the USSR drug addiction was considered antisocial, and it was severely punished. Moreover, use of addictive drugs was harshly controlled in the countries which had become the powerful ideological adversaries of the West: Germany, Italy, and Japan.

During World War II consumption of illicit drugs reached a nadir as the disruption of international transportation also disorganized the drug traffic. Additional restrictive legislation was enacted. Legal cultivation of opium poppies in the United States was regulated by the Opium Poppy Control Act of 1942. Penalties were increased, and synthetic narcotics were placed under federal regulation.

During the campaign against Germany in 1944–45, cocaine or morphine addiction was never a problem among the three million allied soldiers led by General Eisenhower in his Crusade to Europe.[54] And yet, I remember, since I was a battalion doctor at the time, morphine-containing disposable syringes were widely distributed in the front lines to the medics and to the combat soldiers who were instructed to use them only in case of painful wounds. Such instructions were strictly followed, and after combat the soldiers returned the unused syringes, "surettes" as they were called.

One may wonder today if America could have won on two fronts the great struggle of the century against tyranny, if the vast majority of its fighting youth, its blue- and white-collar workers, its professionals, its intellectuals had not been drug-free.

With the end of the war there was an upsurge in addiction, and in 1951 and 1956 Congress enacted legislation requiring mandatory minimum sentences of two years for convicted traffickers.[55] The death penalty was allowed in instances of heroin sales to minors.[56]

This national legislation was reinforced by the International Single Convention on Narcotic Drugs held under the aegis of the United Nations in New York in 1961. The purpose of this Convention was to embody in a single treaty all of the previous international agreements and protocols for control of those drugs having a large potential for abuse. Anslinger headed the American delegation, which also included two seasoned pharmacologists, Dr. Nathan Eddy and Dr. Harry Isbell.[57] Signing parties are obliged to limit the production, manufacture, export, import, distribution of, trade in, use, and possession of, drugs covered by the Convention. The only permitted uses were for medical and scientific purposes. The drugs include, in addition to opium, coca leaves and all of their known derivatives and the flowering or fruiting tops of the cannabis plant.

The inclusion of cannabis in the Convention followed a recommendation of the World Health Organization[58] which had advised the U.S. Commission on Narcotics that "cannabis preparations are practically obsolete and there is no justification for their medical use." The inclusion of cannabis in the Single Convention marked the drug as an illicit substance to be subjected to national and international control, and was the final victory for Anslinger, the Federal Bureau of Narcotics, and all spokesmen for the Progressive movement who had fought for over a half century to reach the goal of banning recreational use of addictive drugs.

However, the Single Convention did not broach the main issue which Porter had sought in vain to introduce at the Second Opium Conference in Geneva: the control at the source in the Far East and South America of the production of the opium poppy and coca leaves. Such control would have required a consensus of the members of the United Nations which was at the time profoundly divided by the cold war. The Single Convention proved to be a pyrrhic victory for the early Progressive American movement and its supporters. In 1967 when the treaty was ratified by the United States Senate, the mood of the country had changed and a whole new outlook was surfacing among some leading intellectuals and opinion-makers. They claimed that repressive methods to contain drug dependence should be replaced by a more humane approach based on a medical model of prevention, treatment, and rehabilitation of the addict. This about-face caught Anslinger and the survivors of the old Progressive guard by surprise. In the last years of their lives, they witnessed the downgrading of the Federal Bureau of Narcotics and the curtailment of its responsibilities, which were assumed by major new bureaucracies that kept growing as addiction to cocaine and other illicit drugs rocketed to unprecedented heights. The studies and warnings of Erlenmeyer, Lewin, and Maier were completely ignored in a new medical and cultural age of liberal drug policy which reopened Pandora's box and led to the great cocaine epidemic of the 1980s.

When one looks back at the immense hardships wrought on millions of people in the world at the turn of the century by the commercial availability of cocaine, and the protracted fight required to control its traffic, it is difficult to comprehend why so many prominent physicians and intellectuals have elected to ignore the lessons of history, in the name of social progress and individual freedom, and have even called for the re-legalization of the most addictive drug known to man.

III

THE UNITED STATES REDISCOVERS COCAINE IN THE 1960S

11

The Re-Opening of Pandora's Box

Anslinger's retirement in 1963 marked the end of a sixty-year period of attempts by the United States to control the non-medical use of addictive drugs primarily by repressive legislation supported by a medical and cultural consensus.

The resulting social taboo against cocaine and other illicit drug use was broken at that time, as a result of profound cultural and economic changes which affected a new generation, seized by a rage to live, driven by a quest for fun which led to a repudiation of past constraints. Popular Freudian theories, often simplified and made to fit current trends, were invoked to account for every aspect of human behavior including drug taking.

Punitive measures could no longer stem the rising tide of discontent, and the pendulum was starting to swing in the opposite direction. A new progressive attitude prevailed among American intellectuals and led them to reconsider previous assumptions about the control and use of addictive drugs. The American Bar Association[1] questioned the principle of mandatory minimum sentences. With the American Medical Association, it established a joint committee in 1961[2] to study the problems created by addictive drugs. This joint committee advocated treatment of addicts in "maintenance" programs instead of punishing them, suggesting that the decision to undertake the cure be voluntary.[3] It also claimed that the new vistas offered by modern medicine and psychiatry could offer a more enlightened solution to addiction than repression and even suggested crime might be prevented by providing addicts with their drug, pointing to "the British model" as an example.

The liberal movement of the 1960's had much in common with the progressive era of the early part of the century. It sponsored measures aimed at enlargement of social and economic justice and at protecting the environment. This reform movement, however, departed from the earlier one by advocating "maintenance" programs for heroin addicts, and even the free availability of addictive drugs, such as cannabis and cocaine, in the name of individual freedom and human rights.

The most articulate spokesman of the movement to reform the laws controlling addictive drugs was Alfred Lindesmith, a university professor of sociology at Indiana University.[4] He believed that regulation rather than prohibition and punishment was the most effective and socially acceptable way to control popular personal vices such as drug abuse. In his view, prohibition creates an illicit traffic that perpetuates the problem, driving it underground and out of control. This result is most apparent in the case of heroin and other opiates; banning their use requires an enforcement bureaucracy dependent on illicit traffic for its very existence. According to Lindesmith (1965), "a comprehensive heroin maintenance program would be a serious or fatal blow to both."[5] In his analysis, Lindesmith erroneously disagreed with the Bureau of Narcotics which claimed that there was a marked decrease in opiate addiction after enactment of the Harrison Act.

Lindesmith looked upon the British system of heroin maintenance as a success, ironically at a time when treatment centers in Britain were beginning methadone use as a substitute for heroin.[6] He also felt that heroin should again be the focus of experimental research in medicine to see if it had a therapeutic use. Except for referring to the current regulatory system for tobacco and alcohol, Lindesmith never clearly defines his idea of regulation. He appears to want to exempt heroin from legal control. Prevention of widespread use of narcotics would then be achieved by the eventual development of some type of social control, a model which has no historical precedent. Heroin is, for Lindesmith, the prototype of the addictive drug, and the same policy should be followed with marijuana and cocaine.

The foundation for Lindesmith's social policy regarding drug addiction was the liberal philosophy of John Stuart Mill[7] as expressed in his famous essay, *On Liberty:* "Over himself, over his own body and mind, the individual is sovereign. In the part which merely concerns himself, his independence is of right, absolute." Other intellectuals, lawyers, and educators also adopted Mill's ideas in the sixties and seventies, which may account for the great success of Lindesmith's book, *The Addict and the Law* (1965). For example, Harry Elmer Barnes, a leading sociologist of the time, praised the book for being "the best general treatment of the subject available in the English language." Written with great clarity and pungency, the book became the liberal establishment's cornerstone for a new reform movement of drug abuse policy.

The new reformers, who dominated American society for the next decades, unlike their predecessors early in the century, associated a permissive attitude towards recreational drug–taking with individual freedom and social progress. Civil libertarians and the American Civil Liberties Union endorsed this policy and succeeded in 1977 in having one of their spokesmen, a psychiatrist, Dr. Peter Bourne, appointed special presidential advisor for drug policy. According to the medical historian David Musto, "the direct access of Bourne to the President and his familiarity with drugs and drug policy made him the government's highest ranking and most influential drug authority in the Nation's history."[8]

Lindesmith's new approach to drug dependence found support among the physicians of the mental health establishment which became the beneficary of massive federal support. By 1969, while the Federal Bureau of Narcotics had an annual budget of $6 million, twice as much as in 1932, the National Institute on Mental Health received in excess of $250 million.[9] The directors of this institute, as well as many of the professors of psychiatry and psychology in academia, professed an attitude quite different from that of the Federal Bureau of Narcotics. They claimed that addiction was a psychological or physical disease and that the medical profession should treat the addicts, first by finding the reasons why they were taking drugs.[10] The notion of addiction as a punishable deviance shifted towards the concept of addiction as a treatable disease and a medical approach to deviance.[11]

The first official departure from the regulatory policies of the previous fifty years occurred at the White Conference on Narcotics and Drug Abuse of 1962 in which Lindesmith participated.[12] Its report distinguishes between the different kinds of addictive drugs and emphasized treatment modalities for addicts. A Presidential Commission in 1963 followed with sweeping recommendations.[13] Relaxation of mandatory minimum sentences, increased appropriations for research into "all aspects of narcotic and drug abuse," and commitment in special centers replaced jailing of convicted addicts.

The dismantling of the Federal Bureau of Narcotics occurred when its functions were transferred to the Justice Department and to the Health, Education, and Welfare Departments (now named the Health and Human Services Department). H.E.W. assumed responsibility for "legitimate" distribution of controlled drugs and research. Justice was responsible for repression of traffic. The medical profession was given the final authority to determine what constitutes legitimate medical treatment and use of narcotic drugs.[14]

Such far-reaching changes shifted the burden of responsibility for control of drug addiction from law enforcement personnel to the medical establishment; they were underpinned by the prevailing belief that the remarkable progress in medicine and psychotherapy of the post-war period had provided physicians, and especially psychiatrists and psychologists, with new methods of treating mental illness and deviant behavior, including drug addiction.

The new medical approach to the control of addiction was, paradoxically, reinforced by the rising use of addictive drugs which started in the sixties, and was attributed by the new reformers to the repressive policies of Anslinger and not to the permissive philosophy of Lindesmith. As the use of illicit drugs rose and addiction, with its associated criminality, soared in the sixties, there was a renewed commitment to medical and psychological treatment. Federal drug regulations retreated from death penalties and mandatory minimum sentences to rely upon "flexible" sentences and addiction maintenance, not only with methadone but also possibly with heroin. The federal government fully supported the medical approach. In 1962 the Supreme Court declared addiction to be a disease, not a crime.[15]

"A program," states Lindesmith,

> which quietly begins to place larger and larger numbers of addicts under the care of doctors would meet with little public disapproval for there is greater public confidence in the medical profession than in the police, lawyers and prosecutors now in charge. It is consistent with our basic ideals of justice, of individual rights, of the proper treatment of the sick. It is progress toward which the United States is moving and for which there is no substitute.[16]

Adoption of Lindesmith's new policy to treat drug addiction medically coincided with the onset of the largest epidemic of illicit drug consumption the United States or any other country in the world has ever experienced — except for China after the Opium Wars. This epidemic developed at a time when the country had reached an unprecedented degree of prosperity and technological supremacy and boasted the highest level of literacy in the world.

The post Korean war generation of the sixties was eager to experiment, disenchanted, rebellious, and no longer motivated by loyalties to family, church, and country, which were considered to be irrelevant vestiges of the past. Freedom and liberation were the catch words of the day. Recreational drug use started with smoking of marijuana, which became widely available and was considered by many physicians and psychiatrists to be an innocuous substance.[17] Regulation was considered to be repressive. There was outrage at the Vietnam War, consumer society, and racial and social inequities. Marijuana smoking became popular as a sign of independent behavior and as one way to express rebellion. Many young people smoked pot without experiencing any ill effects and grew doubtful of its long term damaging and habit-forming properties. Many of these young experimenters felt victimized by erratically enforced repressive legislation.

The taboo against the consumption of illicit substances was broken when prestigious educators candidly accepted the trivialisation of recreational marijuana use. Among them, the famed anthropologist Margaret Mead claimed that "marijuana did not have any harmful physical effects, that it was less dangerous than alcohol and cigarettes and that it should be legalized and sold to any one over the age of 16."[18] The American student population seemed to endorse this view, since a 1969 survey conducted on nine campuses in the western United States reported that 16 to 20% of the students used the drug, and the highest incidence of use was among medical students. Not many of their teachers objected.[19] Numerous books and publications claimed that marijuana was a mild intoxicant and should be legalized, and that the "health sciences had the obligation to guide our society in the judicious use of marijuana" (Lesse, 1971).[20] Some of the most popular volumes were *The Marijuana Smokers* (1970)[21] by the New York State University professor of sociology, Eric Goode; *Marijuana,*

The New Prohibition (1971)[22] by Stanford University professor of law John Kaplan; and *Marijuana Reconsidered* (1971) by Harvard University professor of psychiatry Lester Grinspoon.[23] A new breed of brilliant young intellectuals gave momentum to the marijuana epidemic. The dissenting voices of veteran psychiatrists or pharmacologists Henry Brill,[24] Nathan Eddy,[25] and Abraham Wikler[26] went unnoticed.

My own book, *Marijuana: Deceptive Weed,* which reported the damaging effects of marijuana on mind and body in a historical context, was panned in reviews written by my own colleagues in medical journals.[27] It became fashionable to claim that marijuana was a harmless substance and that one had to learn how to use it like alcohol in a responsible fashion.

In this climate, the United Nations' Single Convention on illicit drugs of 1961 was given scant attention. And yet, its recommendation that the possession of cannabis be considered a punishable offense was signed by President Lyndon Johnson in 1967, and became the law of the land; but nobody in the media mentioned the new legislation which they apparently considered anachronistic.

By contrast, the First Report of the National Commission on Marijuana and Drug Abuse (1972) gave an added momentum to the drug epidemic.[28] The conclusion of the voluminous report recommended "decriminalization of private possession . . . [and] use or distribution of small amounts (one ounce) of marijuana." At the same time it recommended a policy of discouragement of use of the drug through "partial prohibition."

While the decriminalization recommendation did not reflect the opinion of the majority of the American people, it did express that of the liberal wing of academia. It was endorsed by the American Bar Association, The National Education Association, The American Public Health Association, and to some degree by the National Council of Churches, not to mention William S. Buckley, the spokesman for American conservatism.

Despite the commission's recommendation, decriminalization of marijuana remained contrary to federal policy. "I oppose the legalization of marijuana," said President Nixon, "and that includes sale, possession and use. I do not believe you can have effective criminal justice based on a philosophy that something is half legal and half illegal."

Although President Nixon rejected the commission's recommendations, the National Organization for the Reform of Marijuana Laws (NORML) hailed them. Founded a year earlier as the brain child of a midwestern lawyer, Keith Stroup, NORML's purpose was to "liberate marijuana," and endorsement of the National Commission's report gave the organization a powerful weapon for its national campaign.[29]

The Marijuana Commission soon went out of business, and its recommendations would have gathered dust had it not been for NORML. Instead, as Stroup and other reformers testified before the courts and state legislatures across America, they made the Marijuana Commission's report their Bible and pushed for the marijuana decriminalization which was enacted in thirteen states.[30] As an expert witness I attended several hearings which took place across the country, not to argue the legal merits of the case but to rebut statements made by my colleagues Norman Zinberg,[31] Lester Grinspoon,[32] and Thomas Ungerleder,[33] who claimed that marijuana use was not damaging to the mental or physical health of most of the millions of American consumers of the drug.

Such a theme, expounded in most of the publications on the subject which appeared in the 1960s and 1970s, was in turn amplified by the media. As a result a new cultural acceptance of illicit drug use started to emerge in America.

12

The Cultural Acceptance of "Recreational" Drug Use in America

Professor Henry Clay Frick of Columbia University has made a listing of the bestselling books written on addictive drugs between 1965 and 1980 for the general public.[1] Forty-seven of them, published in hard cover and paperback by some of the most prestigious publishing houses, openly advocated the social acceptance of addictive drugs while minimizing their damaging effects. The total number of copies, which exceeded five million, could be found in book stores and libraries all over the country.

We have already mentioned the impact of the volumes written by Professors Kaplan and Grinspoon, both published in 1971, and which advocated the legalization of marijuana. These two books were followed in 1972 by Brecher's *Licit and Illicit Drugs*[2] under the aegis of "Consumers Union." "Consumers Union," which publishes a widely-read periodical dedicated to the impartial protection of consumers' interests, was the first to emphasize the health risks of tobacco smoking. It is highly regarded and read by, among others, community leaders, trade unionists, and reporters. The author of *Licit and Illicit Drugs* was a veteran journalist and medical writer. This 623-page compendium, which has minimal pharmaceutical and scientific input, recommends "methadone and other narcotic maintenance including heroin for heroin addicts . . . [and] the immediate repeal of all federal laws governing the growing, processing, transportation, sale, possession and use of marijuana, and the parallel repeal of existing marijuana laws by each of the fifty states." In effect, the United States was to denounce the United Nations' single convention in order to legalize the sale of marijuana in America.

The influence of *Licit and Illicit Drugs* on American public opinion was considerable. It was widely and favorably reviewed by preeminent lay and professional journals including *The New York Times* and *The New England Journal of Medicine.* The seal of approval given to this book by such prestigious publications, coupled with extensive advertising, resulted in sales which exceeded 200,000 copies.

While *Licit and Illicit Drugs* was considered by many as a reference text, it contains very little accurate scientific data, and merely presents to the general public a slanted and permissive viewpoint about drug use and abuse. A similar viewpoint was formulated a few years later for the intellectual community by the Drug Abuse Council in its final report, "Facts about Drug Abuse." Both texts gave additional momentum to the drug culture. Another book which had a considerable impact on public opinion was *Ganja in Jamaica* by Rubin and Comitas (1976).[3] It concluded that the heavy consumption of cannabis in Jamaica does not produce any physical or mental impairment, and that the "ganja" habit has a favorable influence on Jamaican society and "motivates" sugar cane farmers. This book, available in mass paperback, became the bible of the drug culture and an often-quoted reference whenever the subject of marijuana came up in the media. Other books published by prestigious publishing houses under titles which clearly described their content and messages included: *The Connoisseur Handbook of Marijuana* by Drake (1971),[4] The Gourmet Coke Book (anonymous),[5] *The Dope Book* by Lieberman (1978),[6] *The Gourmet Guide to Grass* by Rosoff (1978),[7] *Psychedelic Baby Reaches Puberty* by Stafford (1971),[8] and *Responsible Drug and Alcohol Use* by Eng (1979).[9] The latter contains "hints for the responsible use of Marijuana" such as, "smoke with friends, clean out the seeds, know your drug, use a water pipe or non-inflammable roach clip, and don't drop ashes or you'll burn holes in your clothes." In 1980 the journalist and reviewer William Novak published *High Culture,* which describes the pervasiveness of marijuana in the lives of Americans.[10]

By contrast, there were only nine books written between 1965 and 1980 for the general public which stressed the biological and social dangers of drugs. Only one of them was available from a publishing house specializing in large paperback editions. The total number of copies published during the 1970s did not exceed 200,000. They were rarely displayed in book stores and could be obtained only in a limited number of school or public libraries. They were outnumbered 50 to 1 by the permissive publications on the subject.

Under the impact of such a massive, one-sided source of "primary" information, the mass media followed suit. All of the books mentioned in Frick's list, which is not even complete, inspired articles in the daily and periodical press as well as discussion on radio and television interviews. Their drug-dismissive and misleading conclusions were replicated in hundreds of thousands of newsletters and pamphlets written by private and government organizations specializing in drug-abuse prevention and education.

Some of the organizations catering to the drug culture selected revealing names for themselves. The "Do It Now Foundation" published numerous pamphlets including a periodical called "Drug Survival News." The pamphlets carry a very clear message: "Since most people experiment with drugs they'd better learn about them and what to do if one gets sick after taking them." In 1980, the "Do it Now Foundation" described itself as one of the nation's largest suppliers of drug-education materials, many of which were purchased by state Drug Abuse and Alcohol agencies and disseminated to school children throughout the country. In one of its pamphlets, "A Realistic Primer for Parents" by Dr. V. Pawlak, "Do it Now" advises parents:

> Marijuana to date (1980) has not been proven physically harmful even in remote ways, . . . and the mild psychological changes that occur in many people are considered to be generally beneficial in nature, and have evolved into what is commonly called "a good place for your head to be."[11]

In 1980 "Do it Now" was listed by the National Institute on Drug Abuse (NIDA) as one of the sources of drug education material for schools. When, under pressure from parents' movment, NIDA dropped "Do it Now" from its resource list, it was consigned to the ranks of all the "illiterati" relentlessly denounced by "Do it Now" because they presented evidence indicating the health hazards of marijuana. Another organization which catered even more directly to the drug culture was STASH, the "Student Association for the Study of Hallucinogens."[12] STASH also preached "chemical survival" to its constituency of high school and university students.

In 1975, publications entirely devoted to drugs and drug users such as *Head, High Times,* and *Stone Age* started to appear on newstands. These slick magazines glamorized the use of cocaine and of marijuana, extolling the heroic lives of the smugglers of "hashish and snow"; they also carried ads from the paraphernalia industry, a burgeoning new American business which rose from an estimated $12 million volume in 1972 to $500 million in 1974 and specialized in the manufacture and sale of all the gadgets and instruments needed for the proper consumption of cannabis or cocaine: these included "kits to make freebase cocaine" which, when smoked, is one of the most addictive and destructive of drugs. A full-page advertisement in *The New York Times* in 1979 claimed 4 million readers for *High Times*.[13] A quotation from William Burroughs, a candid authority on the subject, gives the best description of this kind of literature (which can be found only in the United States and is banned in Canada):

> Junk is their ultimate merchandise — the junk merchant does not sell his product to the consumer, he sells the consumer to the product. He never improves his merchandise, he degrades the client.[14]

One could not expect the mass media to take a stand counter to the popular groundswell of the new reform movement and its surrogates which advocated a more liberal and less punitive approach towards the use of marijuana and of other addictive drugs.

In 1970, a *Newsweek* cover story (Sept. 7) featured the movement in "Marijuana, Time to Change the Law," and in 1971 *The New York Times Book Review* published a laudatory front-page review of Grinspoon's book, *Marijuana Reconsidered* (1971), which advocated legalization of the drug and which was dubbed "the best dope on pot so far."[15] Books which expressed a contrary viewpoint were not reviewed by the *Times,* according to a study by a senior United States Senate analyst, David Martin, in 1981.

That same year an editorial in *The New York Times* advocated the "British model" of supplying heroin to heroin addicts.[16] The media reflect and amplify public opinion. Their influence in reporting the sensational is well-known and is clearly analyzed by the French sociologist Emile Durkheim, who cautioned at the end of the 19th century against the danger inherent in reporting murders or suicide in a neutral fashion — a fashion, he said, which might excite rather than "neutralize individual propensities." "If a society," writes Durkheim (in 1897), "is in a state of moral disarray, its uncertainty reveals itself when, faced with immoral acts, it treats them with an involuntary indulgence which tones down their very immorality. Then does example become a threat, not so much as an example but because of social tolerance and indifference."[17]

The gist of Durkheim's comments is that the reporting of antisocial acts such as murder or suicide by the media must have a negative connotation in order to avoid a snowball effect, and this implies a moral judgment. A little less than a century later, the media were reluctant to make a value judgment on drug abuse. Was it because such a denunciation might have threatened the individual's freedom of choice, or ran counter to a trend of the time? In any case, the neutral attitude adopted by the media to events organized by the drug culture such as rallies, "smoke-ins," and rock concerts where drug consumption became an integral part of the fun reinforced the popularity of such happenings.

High Times, a knowledgeable source in this matter, wrote in its October 1977 issue:

> The media attention [was] leading to the mass turn ons of the mid sixties . . . and a wave of media publicity about the gentleness of this mass turn on resulted in an even larger gathering in San Francisco's Golden Gate Park in January, 1967. An estimated 10,000 turned on.

During the turbulent seventies and early eighties only one of the mass-circulated monthly lay publications remained staunchly on the side of the early reformers and refused to ondone the social acceptance of marijuana and of other illicit drugs. *The Reader's Digest,* which since its inception has striven to express and defend the basic values of grassroots America and "The American Way of Life," regularly published articles, many written by veteran reporter Peggy Mann, which warned against the health hazards of illicit drug consumption. This publication might be looked down upon by the highbrows of Western intelligentsia. However the far sighted policy of the editors of *The Reader's Digest* in combatting the trivialization of illicit drugs in America and the trend of the time should be recognized now that it has been vindicated. It took courage and wisdom to counteract all of the misleading information which was streaming out of the mass media. In this instance, for years the lonely voice of *The Reader's Digest,* while it did not reach the silent and hallowed halls of academia, could still be heard by the people of America.

While the minds and hearts of young people in the sixties and seventies were receiving, through the media, Dr. Timothy Leary's message to "turn on" with the help of marijuana and L.S.D., a similar appeal was being delivered by some of their favorite musicians. The lyrics of the musicians were amplified by the sounds of drums, electric guitars, or organs amid flashing multicolored lights. The drug-oriented songs of the sixties had a major impact on the youth of America and western Europe. One cannot underestimate the effects on young people of "pop music," which has become for many a modern cult while pop performers are their new idols. Folk music "rock and roll" express in a noisy fashion the enthusiastic vitality of youth engaging a great time.[18]

Rock and roll productions are entirely oriented towards the teenage and young adult market of teenagers which can absorb 100 million discs a year. A number–one record on the Hit Parade list will be purchased by more than half a million youngsters in the U.S., and will be subsequently released in western Europe. In addition, a successful record will be programmed on jukeboxes all across the American and European continents and played innumberable times on radio stations around the world.

The first popular song to carry a veiled message about a drug which "lets your mind roll on" (marijuana) was a folk song, "Walk Right" (1962). Then came "Puff the Magic Dragon," and in 1965 the famous "Mr. Tambourine Man," written by Bob Dylan, which combined a rock and roll background with folk lyrics, started the vogue of "psychedelic music." The message delivered in its content and performance suggested the drugged state and experience. As reported by Taqui, "Many of the most popular songs had a tone and content which implied a drug-centered meaning" and hence could trigger drug-oriented behavior in the brains of the youth exposed to the song.

The following records, which were international hits, are good examples of drug-centered songs which reached tens of millions of listeners:

Eight Miles High (1966), *Along Comes Mary* (1966), *Acupolco Gold* (Mexican marijuana) (1967), *The Pusher* (1968), and the famous songs of the Beatles, *Happiness is a Warm Gun* (the gun is, in drug jargon, a syringe), *Yellow Submarine* (the submarine is a capsule containing amphetamines or any other drug), and *Sergeant Pepper*. The Beatles song which most clearly alludes to L.S.D. (lysergic acid diethylamide — "acid" — a drug that produces hallucinations), *Lucy in the Sky with Diamonds,* is one of the biggest selling records of all times. And in order to clear away any possible ambiguity, when *Sergeant Pepper* reached the sales rack, the Beatles admitted they had used L.S.D., and their free use of marijuana was no secret to any of their fans.

After *Sergeant Pepper* the theme of drugs in rock and roll became prevalent among all pop musicians, and their youthful audiences did not hesitate to smoke marijuana or take acid in order to "tune in." Many rock concerts after the famous Woodstock became "smoke-ins." *Mind Excursion, Flying High, Stoned Soul Picnic, Comin' Down, Girl Called Sandoz,* and *Get Off on My Cloud* are just a few of the most suggestive titles.

Following the lyrics extolling the virtues of marijuana and L.S.D., those chanting the unequalled cocaine experience appeared first timidly in 1966 with Laura Nyro. Her song *Buy and Sell* ("cocaine and quiet beers") was followed by *Getting Off the Poverty Train* ("something better than getting off on sweet cocaine"). In 1970 two major rock groups sang the praise of cocaine: The Rolling Stones with *Let it Bleed* ("when you need a little coke") and the Grateful Dead's *Casey Jones* ("driving that train high on cocaine") and *Trucking* ("living on reds, Vitamin C, and cocaine"). In 1971 Jefferson Airplane sang "Earth mother children here, ripped on coke and feeling dandy," and the Rolling Stones followed the same year with "Sister morphine and sweet cousin cocaine."[19] As Grinspoon states, "The ideal large scale cocaine consumer for financial, professional and cultural reasons is a rock musician."[20]

Rolling Stones, the journal of the rock and pop culture, headlined in 1971 "A flash in the pan, a pain in the nose." This article on cocaine claimed that the new drug was already responsible for "wasting a number of top musical names."[21]

Illicit drug use became a part of rock and roll entertainment as many rock celebrities adopted the marijuana or cocaine habits, believing that the drug experience was a meaningful expansion of consciousness leading to the discovery of new worlds. A few of them, like John Lennon in Japan, were arrested for drug offenses, and some, like Jimmy Hendrix, succumbed to fatal overdose of heroin.

Drug-centered lyrics could never have reached the public without being promoted by record companies and radio stations which were overwhelmed by popular demand for the records of the Beatles and the Rolling Stones and could not forgo the handsome profits which they brought in. A permissive society which has removed the cultural taboos about drug use cannot expect the record industry to reinstate them by refusing to disseminate drug-oriented songs.

All of these songs, composed and executed by the heroes of millions of adolescents, contributed markedly to the spreading of the drug culture. Responsible adults shrugged their shoulders most of the time, unaware of the potential damaging effect of such music, which left them indifferent but enticed their children into smoking marijuana or snorting cocaine. Few parents were aware of the inherent damage of disharmonic rock music on the brain of the listener, as demonstrated in experimental studies.[22]

The film industry, which both reflects and reinforces prevailing trends in society, also started to include cocaine use in its productions. In 1970 *The Private Life of Sherlock Holmes* featured the famous private eye self-administering the drug. One of the most popular films of 1971 was *Easy Rider* which makes heroes out of cocaine dealers and users; it was a greater box office success than *A Man for all Seasons.*[23] In 1972, the most entertaining movie, *Superfly,* features a cocaine dealer as its hero who outwits the corrupt agents in charge of drug enforcement and lives handsomely from his drug profits.

All through the sixties and seventies, at a marked crescendo the American people and especially the young were exposed to a steady visual and auditory bombardment emanating from the printed and spoken word, the press, radio, movie, and television — music and song which overtly or subliminally alluded to the drug experience. The available statistics abundantly indicate that such a pervasive exposure to the drug culture had an important influence on drug consumption. Within twenty years, America became the greatest consumer of illicit drugs in the world, and especially of the most dangerous of them all, cocaine. To quote Ashley, an amateur historian of that era, "The police and the media had given it such an incredible reputation, that it would hardly have been human not to try it."

13

After Marijuana: Heroin and Cocaine

The smoking of marijuana and consumption of hallucinogens such as LSD were overshadowed in the late sixties by the use of heroin and cocaine. The number of addicts self-administering heroin intravenously, which had stabilized at around 50,000 between 1930 and 1950, reached epidemic proportions, especially in large urban centers. In 1968 it was estimated to be over one half million, a figure comparable on a per capita basis to the number of opiate and cocaine addicts at the turn of the century when the population of the United States was only half as large. Death by overdose exceeded one thousand per year. Criminality associated with drug dependence increased as the number of addicts soared.

Congress responded to this onslaught of drug abuse by enacting new legislation. Law enforcement was streamlined: in 1968, the Federal Bureau of Narcotics was placed in the Department of Justice and became the Bureau of Narcotics and Dangerous Drugs, later renamed the Drug Enforcement Agency. Its budget in 1972 was $60 million, compared to the $4 million expended by the Federal Bureau of Narcotics in 1962.

In 1966 Congress passed the Narcotic Addict Rehabilitation Act which provided medical treatment as an alternative to prison and dropped the mandatory minimum sentences for heroin traffic adopted a decade earlier.[1] The Comprehensive Drug Abuse and Prevention Act of 1970[2] differentiated between various types of drugs and restated the interstate commerce regulations as the constitutional basis for drug control. It also created the National Commission of Marijuana and Drug Abuse, increased enforcement personnel, defined offenses, and set penalties.

In 1972, the National Institute on Drug Abuse (NIDA)[3] was established to develop and conduct comprehensive health, education, training, and research programs for the prevention and treatment of drug abuse and the rehabilitation of drug abusers. All of this new legislation reiterated the basic U.S. policy of excluding addictive drugs, so damaging to the individual and to society, from the flow of American commerce. But for the first time provisions were adopted emphasizing rehabilitation of addicts with methadone maintenance programs as well as psychiatric treatment. Such provisions gave back to physicians, and more so to psychiatrists, a prominent role in the "treatment" of drug addicts, and a greater voice in the formulation of drug abuse programs and policy.

The seventies were marked by the extensive use of drugs by all segments of American society, particularly adolescents, and by the emergence of a drug culture unprecedented in modern times. One of this era's most salient features besides the well-orchestrated campaign to decriminalize marijuana was the development of large–scale heroin treatment programs using methadone maintenance.[4]

Methadone, an opiate synthetic derivative which can be taken by mouth once a day, has been given to heroin addicts as a substitute for heroin, a drug which has to be injected into the veins four times a day in order to avoid withdrawal symptoms. This method, pioneered by Dr. Vincent Dole of the Rockefeller Institute,[5] decreases the demand for heroin; but methadone is an addictive drug derived from morphine. It must be given under supervision to avoid illegal diversion, and has to be associated with supportive measures requiring a well-trained and devoted staff.

In spite of wide–scale experimentation, methadone maintenance did not become the "magic bullet" it was purported to be by some of its proponents.[6] Between June, 1971, and June, 1973, 100,000 treatments slots were funded by federal and state appropriations in every major urban center. The $350 million federal budget allotted for 1973 remained at approximately the same annual level through 1980. If one adds to this figure $150 million from state, local, and private sources, half a billion dollars were spent every year during that period for treatment and rehabilitation of addicts, primarily heroin addicts.

Treatment of heroin addiction therefore achieved the status of a major American industry in the seventies. Many problems arose in the course of methadone programs: diversion of the drug to the black market; a drop-out rate of half of those entering the program; a lack of qualified staff to restore the addict to society; and a high incidence of alcohol, marijuana, or cocaine use among those remaining on maintenance, which indicated that the substitution of methadone for heroin did not eliminate drug-seeking behavior. Conflicts arose between physicians and federal policy–makers.[7] The former believed that life-long maintenance on methadone should be considered for hard-core addicts, while the latter believed that methadone should be used for only a limited period in order to "detoxify" addicts and orient them towards a drug-free life. However, administration of methadone is preferable to the injecting of heroin and the possible infections with the AIDS virus associated with this procedure. The large-scale experimental use of chemicals to "treat" heroin addiction proved discouraging. Even the use of a nonaddictive substance such as clonidine,[8] an antihypertensive drug, which suppresses the withdrawal symptom of the opiate addicts, did not result in a "cure" for the addict. Dr. Mark Gold who initiated this therapy states that it must be reinforced with psychotherapy and other rehabilitative measures. For some addicts the prospect of a comfortable symptom-free withdrawal leads to a recurrent cycle of addiction rather than to a commitment to a demanding rehabilitation program essential for a long-term recovery and drug-free life.

Methadone maintenance runs counter to the conviction of advocates in the early reform movement who stated that "addiction should be stopped, not catered to." In addition, the lack of overall effectiveness of this treatment dashed the great hope of the social reformers who had hoped that new medical intervention would rapidly become available to cure heroin addiction. But the new drug reformers were not ready to admit, as did the proponents of the Harrison Act, that "there is no treatment of heroin addiction which leads to abstinence in more than a fraction of attempts.[9] This statement also applies to cocaine addiction, which is even more difficult to interrupt than the heroin habit, as many of the physicians of the turn of the century had already reported. But their American counterparts of today have failed to recognize this fact and have repeated the same errors of judgment committed by Freud in 1885.

While the consumption of heroin after the dramatic increase noted in the sixties had stabilized at half a million users, in the mid-seventies other illicit drugs were consumed at an increasing rate. This was especially true for cocaine, which in 1974 was recognized in the *New York Times* magazine as the "champagne of drugs."[10] This piece had been preceded by a flurry of medical and lay publications which described the beneficial effects of cocaine on mood and behavior while underestimating its health hazards and addictive power. Richard Woodley's portrayal of a successful Harlem cocaine dealer,[11] published in 1971, was followed in 1974 by "About Harry Townes."[12] This novel, written by Bruce Friedman, describes the use of cocaine by an upper class gentleman for whom the drug has become an integral part of his life. Ashley's popular book *Cocaine. Its History, Uses, and Effects*,[13] published in 1975, claims that the drug has been wrongly disqualified from society "by moral outrage or scientific ignorance" and calls for its "relegalization." This volume was hailed as "admirable" by the *Washington Post* and as "a balanced, lucid and common sense study" by the *Publisher's Weekly*.

> "By 1972," writes Ashley, "cocaine was no novelty, and especially not to the affluent types who had been smoking marijuana for a few years. These people, for whom grass had replaced the predinner martini, were buyers in the illicit drug market and naturally met up with cocaine. They are garment district executives, models, designers, salesmen, admen, doctors, lawyers, bankers, professors, writers—indeed they simply represented a healthy cross-section of those who lead the good life in America's major cities. And just as at an earlier time they had been introduced to marijuana by a friend, they were now introduced to cocaine. Marijuana hadn't hurt them so they saw no good reason not to try cocaine."[14]

The *Gourmet Coke Book,* though written by an anonymous author, became a best-seller.[15] Mortimer's laudatory book *History of Coca,* published in 1902, was reprinted by the And/Or Press in 1974.[16] This volume could have been entitled *In Praise of Coca,* expanding as it does in great detail on the beneficial effects of the leaf as described by Freud in *Uber Coca.* The latter text was reprinted in numerous publications. All of these authors distinguished between "recreational use" which could be controlled by most consumers, like Freud, and which was the usual pattern in the U.S., and chronic, heavy usage which was rare and seemed to belong to the distant past. They all claimed that the drug did not induce "physical dependence," tolerance, or withdrawal symptoms and was not addictive. Dr. Peter Bourne, who became the drug adviser to President Carter, wrote an article entitled "The Great Cocaine Myth" and stated: "Cocaine is probably the most benign of illicit drugs currently in widespread use. At least as strong a case could be made for legalizing it as for legalizing marijuana—short acting—about 15 minutes, not physically addicting, and acutely pleasurable—cocaine has found increasing favor at all socio-economic levels in the last year."[17]

A standard psychiatry textbook[18] published in 1980 states: "Used no more than two or three times a week, cocaine creates no serious problem. . . . At present chronic cocaine use does not usually present a medical problem." Lester Grinspoon, one of the authors of this statement, had expressed essentially the same opinion about marijuana ten years earlier. And in 1975 he wrote, with J.P. Bakalar, a monographs on cocaine which justifies its recreational use.[19] This is one of the most thoroughly documented monographs on the subject (except for the pharmacological properties of the drug on brain and body). The book discusses most of the early reports of Erlenmeyer, Lewin, and Maier, which describe the addictive and damaging properties of cocaine. However, the conclusions and warnings of these older authors are dismissed by Grinspoon and Bakalar, who still condone the recreational, responsible use of this drug by physicians and their patients. The following quotations reflect the permissive philosophy of Grinspoon:

> There remains a large area in which medicine and recreation, diseases and problems of living overlap. . . . What a physician does when he prescribes a tranquilizer (Valium) is not fundamentally different from what a layman does when he prescribes (to himself) a beer, a marijuana cigarette or a sniff of cocaine. . . . Physicians can be prudent and sparing in their use of drugs without relying on an unworkable conceptual puritanism as a justification. . . . It is arbitrary to pronounce medicinal use of a given drug good, and recreational use bad, if the only basis for the distinction between medicine and pleasure is the institutional authority of the physician himself.

All of this loose rhetoric ignores the lessons of basic pharmacology and clinical medicine, by placing in the same category coffee, marijuana, tranquilizers, and cocaine. Lacking this scientific knowledge, Grinspoon and Bakalar overlook the unique inherent properties of cocaine to impair brain bio-chemical mechanisms which underlie all of man's thought pro-cesses. Their integrity is essential for the exercise of human reason, judgment and "free" will, a fact which Grinspoon and Bakalar seem unable to understand.

The general opinion about the relative safety of cocaine was so prevalent in the Boston area, that circuit judge Elwood McKenney of Roxbury, Massachusetts, ruled in 1977 that cocaine was "an irrational addition to federal and state nar-cotics laws, resulting from generations of ignorance, from myths connected with the drug." As a result, a man arrested for possession of the drug was released. The judge based his opin-ion on the testimony of expert witnesses Dr. Norman Zin-berg[20] and Dr. Andrew Weil[21] from Harvard University. No evidence was presented during the trial showing adverse reac-tions to cocaine.

The possible role of marijuana use in the spread of co-caine usage was documented in a 1982 study by the social researchers Clayton and Voss.[22] These authors established a very significant statistical association between prior marijuana smoking and subsequent cocaine use: data supporting the link-age between marijuana and cocaine usage is more than ten times greater than the evidence of linkage between tobacco smoking and lung cancer. A very similar linkage was docu-mented by these same authors between heroin use and prior marijuana exposure. These studies confirm those previously performed in 1975 by Professor Denise Kandel of Columbia University.[23]

In September of 1975 a White Paper on Drug Abuse was presented to President Ford by representatives of eleven federal departments concerned by this problem. Cocaine was consid-ered as a drug less dangerous than amphetamines and heroin and it was recommended that less emphasis be placed by the Drug Enforcement Agency on curtailing cocaine traffic and that it concentrate more on the heroin trade in Mexico.[24]

In the late seventies, as cocaine became more socially acceptable, more freely available, and liberally used, the side effects observed a hundred years ago among cocaine users were reported again: marked tolerance, compulsive drug consump-tion, paranoid psychosis, and sudden death caused by heavy "recreational use" of the drug reported by Wetli in 1979.[25] But the numbers of these reports were not large enough, given the numbers of consumers, to create serious alarm among the new specialists on cocaine dependence working in the hallowed halls of academia or in the National Institute on Drug Abuse.

The unprecedented call for the social acceptance of cocaine recreational use was supported by American physicians and academics who elected to break with the medical and social consensus which had prevailed concerning the addictive and destructive potential of this drug.

Could it be for such reasons that today the U.S., in spite of its unequalled leadership in the medical sciences, is in the throes of a cocaine epidemic of proportions unprecedented in the history of mankind?

14

Cocaine, The Intellectual Establishment, and the Parents of America

The desire to change drug laws in order to satisfy the demand for greater drug availability in society was apparent not only to the many advocates of recreational drug use but also to the leaders of America's most prestigious foundations.

In 1970 the trustees of the Ford Foundation commissioned two Washington lawyers, Patricia Wald (who later became a circuit judge) and Peter Hutt, to undertake an in-depth survey of the problem of drug abuse. The purpose was to research what private foundations might contribute to the understanding and solution of this problem. Wald and Hutt's report was called "Dealing with Drug Abuse." In it they wrote:

> It is of fundamental importance that man has and will inevitably continue to have potentially dangerous drugs at his disposal, which he may either use properly or abuse, and that neither the availability of these drugs nor the temptation to abuse them can be eliminated. Therefore, *the fundamental objective of a modern drug-abuse program must be to help the public learn to understand these drugs and how to cope with their use in the context of everyday life.* An approach emphasizing suppression of all drugs or repression of all drug users will only contribute to national problems.[1]

By the stroke of a pen, two lawyers were dismissing the policy wisely and painstakingly formulated over a half century, that had, when implemented, first rolled back and then controlled cocaine addiction in the Western world.

The "modern drug abuse program" which was advocated merely reflected the liberal drug policy earlier advocated by Alfred Lindesmith,[2] and it was similarly based on the assumption that men are motivated by reason alone and may therefore be taught the responsible use of addictive drugs. This opinion set the stage for a major policy shift. In order to carry out this shift, the federal government and the United Nations had to be bypassed. Therefore Wald and Hutt made the following recommendation:

> There is an urgent need for effective nongovernmental leadership toward a more reasoned approach to drug abuse in this country. A void exists that we believe can be filled by the creation of a new Drug Abuse Council. In our best judgment the Council could successfully exert this leadership and could have a substantial and beneficial impact on drug abuse in this country.[3]

In effect they were recommending that an independent, private organization with the financial means to influence public opinion and advocate a liberal drug policy be instituted.

The trustees of the Ford Foundation endorsed the creation of the Drug Abuse Council with a $7.5 million grant. Three other foundations, Carnegie, Kaiser, and Commonwealth, pledged an additional $2.5 million. Further funds came from the Equitable Life Assurance Society, the United Methodist Church, the City of Phoenix, and the United States State Department.[4]

The Council was formed in January, 1972, for a five-year period. The roster of its Board of Directors, reading like *Who's Who in America,*[5] listed representatives from universities and leaders from the business and legal professions. None had any experience in the field of drug dependence, however.

Dr. Thomas Bryant was selected by the Ford Foundation to be president of the Council. He was a psychiatrist who also held a law degree and had some experience in the federal antipoverty program, but none in the field in which he was to chart new policy. As recalled by Patrick Andersen,

> In mid-1973 Bryant joined the National Organization for the Repeal of Marijuana Laws (NORML), as a member of the advisory board. He also made Stroup, the Director of NORML, a $200-a-month consultant to the Council—not an insignificant amount of money in those days. Most important, the Council began giving grants of up to $30,000 a year to NORML's "nonpolitical" spinoff, the Center for the Study of Non-Medical Drug Use. Money given to the Center was used for such "nonpolitical" purposes as lawsuits, publishing costs, and the like, which of course freed other NORML money for its political activities. Indirectly, the Council was subsidizing

NORML's political and legislative program, helping NORML do things that the Council thought needed doing but that it legally could not do. The alliance benefited both parties. It gave NORML money, credibility, and increased access to the respectable scientists and policy makers who clustered around the Council. For Bryant, alliance with NORML was a move to the left. As Stroup saw it, NORML had, in effect, become the political arm of the Drug Abuse Council. It was a delicate arrangement, given the tax laws and the Ford Foundation's sensitivity to criticism that it was subsidizing liberal political causes, but it was one that for several years was crucial to NORML's success.[6]

Dr. Bryant assembled a staff of younger academics, trained in law, sociology, journalism, and political science. None of them had any expertise in pharmacology, the neurosciences, internal medicine, or epidemiology. Medical scientists were not needed by the Council, which had been given the political task of justifying the liberal drug policy endorsed by the Ford Foundation, a policy based on four assumptions: The widespread inescapable availability of drugs; the desire of people to use them; the failure of the criminal justice system to prevent their use; and the possibility of using drugs in a "responsible fashion."[7]

The Drug Abuse Council embarked on an ambitious program of grants, contracts, internal studies, fellowships, and special publications, many of the endorsing "decriminalization" of marijuana. Six years later, in 1980, after spending its $10 million, the Council published its final report; *Facts About Drug Abuse*. In reality, this volume contains few facts, but numerous opinions, and omits major parts of the scientific and historical record on the subject.

The partial and selective recording of "facts" is most apparent in the Council's treatment of the decriminalization of marijuana. Central to their arguments in favor of this policy is the assertion that decriminalization will not increase use of the drug. The surveys made by the Council in Oregon and California[8] to prove this hypothesis are fragmentary and incomplete, as pointed out by Rusche,[9] they also conflict with the systematic epidemiologic surveys of Professor Johnston[10] from the University of Michigan. The latter indicate that daily marijuana use among high school seniors in the U.S. increased from 6% to 10.8% between 1975 and 1979. These figures, available to the Council, were not mentioned in its report.

The Council, not content with recommending freer availability of marijuana, called for similar measures for cocaine.

> The law has classified cocaine as a serious drug of abuse. Yet
> despite substantial efforts by some researchers to prove this
> contention its moderate use does not appear to result in signifi-
> cant personal or social harm other than that of the effects of the
> criminal process on detected users.[11]

This conclusion was based on the following scientific surveys made by the drug experts of the Council:

> Medical experts generally agree that cocaine produces few ob-
> servable health consequences in its users. . . . Recent Ameri-
> can psychiatric and sociological studies have failed to substanti-
> ate the view that repeated cocaine use leads to physiological
> dependence or tolerance. . . . In this respect American cocaine
> use appears to resemble a common pattern in alcohol use in
> which fine wines or liquors are reserved for other than ordinary
> consumption.[12]

The Council's conclusion? "By adhering to an unrealistic
goal of total abstinence from the use of illicit drugs, op-
portunities to *encourage* responsible drug using behavior are
missed." The final report also notes: "Since the creation of the
Drug Abuse Council in 1972, more Americans appear to be
using more psychoactive substances. Drug use and misuse
have become the most compelling realities of American Society."[13] That this result might have been brought about by the
very policies supported by the Drug Abuse Council is a possibility that cannot be easily dismissed. However, the Drug
Abuse Council should not be held entirely responsible for the
social acceptance of marijuana and cocaine in American Society. The Council was merely amplifying a cultural trend which
emerged in the sixties with the student revolt and the new
reform movement led by the medical and psychiatric establishment that we have described. But the prestige of the foundations which created and supported the Council added considerable weight to the drug policies formulated by the latter and
which were subsequently endorsed by the new reformers of
academia and the media who found new arguments to advocate the relegalization of illicit drugs and their responsible use.

No other book did more to bring this message of the Drug
Abuse Council to the public than *Chocolate to Morphine* by
Andrew Weil, M.D., and Winifred Rosen.[14] Published in
1983 by Houghton Mifflin, this handsomely illustrated and

well written book is authored by a physician (graduate of Harvard) and, at times, fervent advocate of psychedelic drug use. His co-author is a young adult novelist, author of more than a dozen books for young people. Both have adopted the premises of the Drug Abuse Council which they formulate in their opening statement: "Drugs are here to stay and history teaches that it is vain to hope that drugs will ever disappear and that any effort to eliminate them from society is doomed to failure."[15] After such a misreading of history Weil and Rosen make two simple recommendations:

> Either to teach young people to satisfy their desires without recourse to drugs, or to teach them how to form good relationships with drugs so that if they choose to use drugs, they will continue to be users and never become abusers. . . . With drugs so available and with children so disposed to experiment with them this teaching is vital. Young people are going to decide for themselves whether to use drugs. The most that responsible adults can hope to do is give children the information that will enable them to use drugs intelligently if they choose to use them at all. . . . A period of experimentation with drugs is today a normal phase of adolescence — a rite of passage — that most children pass through unscathed.[16]

And finally, "there are no good or bad drugs — only good or bad users of drugs."[17] The authors go on to describe how to use addictive drugs responsibly, accumulating major pharmacological and historical omissions and errors. A few examples:

> "The worst features of heroin addiction are due to the social situation in which they are taken, rather than to the pharmacological effects of opiates,"[18] which, he claims, help addicts to resist disease.[19]
> "Unlike alcohol, marijuana does not invariably depress reflexion [sic] and reaction times."[20]
> "By outlawing coca, laws have encouraged a vast black market in cocaine."[21]
> Weil's recommendation: "Take stimulants purposefully and do not combine stimulants with depressants."[22]

The book was widely used throughout the country by drug counselors and in college courses on drug dependence. The publisher found psychiatry professor Norman Zinberg, tennis professional Arthur Ashe, and many other specialists and prominent personalities to recommend his book "to young and older readers, parents and teachers alike."

As long as such misinformation is widely disseminated it will not be possible to restore the social refusal of cocaine and other addictive drugs, a refusal which throughout history has allowed the United States and many other nations to protect their societies against the trivialization of drug use.

The conclusions of the Drug Abuse Council did not only influence popular writers. The National Institute on Drug Abuse (NIDA), which had to chart a policy on drug dependence for the nation, could not ignore the views expressed by the intellectual establishment on the acceptance of "recreational drug use," including cocaine.

From its inception NIDA was dominated by young psychiatrists from Harvard and the University of Chicago,[23] who did not take the time to consult the older authors but had been influenced by the proponents of the new medical model of drug addiction put forth by Lindesmith in the sixties: The drug addict is a sick person requiring medical treatment, not a delinquent to be prosecuted. The main goal of NIDA was a scientific investigation of the causes of drug dependence so as to eradicate them through new strategies. They believed eventually the scientist would find a magic bullet to cure addiction. However, NIDA, unlike the National Heart Institute, was not integrated into the existing prestigious National Institutes of Health headed by outstanding scientists and devoted to medical research, but rather into a newly-created federal bureaucracy, the Alcohol, Drug Abuse and Mental Health Administration (ADAMHA). ADAMHA comprised, in addition to NIDA, two other institutes: the National Institute on Mental Health and the Nation Institute on Alcoholism. All three organizations presented as a common feature the predominance of psychiatrists, psychologists, and social scientists in their upper echelons. The budget of ADAMHA rose from $450 million in 1975 to one and a half billion dollars in 1987.[24] Paralleling this approximately three-fold increase in ADAMHA's budget, the number of cocaine users increased five-fold from 4 to 20 million during the same period: the size of the drug epidemic was rising still faster than the budget of ADAMHA. And yet the bulk of the funds were allocated to treatment and to prevention programs. NIDA–sponsored research in the field of drug dependence was mostly performed under the aegis of universities and at the Addiction Research Center which had been moved from Lexington to Baltimore. This research was not goal-oriented towards systematically establishing the toxic effects of cocaine on vital physiological functions. Some grants supported studies of limited biochemical changes in isolated tissues and from which no clear cut conclusion could be derived concerning the acute or chronic impairment effects of cocaine. However, this work could be silently pursued in the ivory tower of universities and by specialized scientists studying very *basic* mechanisms and who were unwilling to enter the public fray. Other grants supported studies of the effects of small doses of cocaine administered to man (cocaine addicts) under controlled laboratory conditions.[25]

These latter studies did not yield any more information than had already been known for a hundred years, but raised serious conceptual objections which will be discussed in Chapter XXIV. Rather than sponsor "open-ended studies" supported by research grants, it would have been more effective for NIDA to distribute its funds in the form of goal-oriented contracts focused on specific topics such as effects of cocaine on the heart, the kidney, the immune system, the liver, and the brain. But it seemed that NIDA was somewhat reluctant to support such studies, which could have given strong arguments to those who opposed the social acceptance of illicit drug use. I had already found this out, along with some of my other colleagues who studied the damaging effects of marijuana on reproductive function or immunity or brain.[26] Reports which indicated the damaging effect of marijuana met with great skepticism and even created public outrage in some cases. And, NIDA was not eager to pursue the support of projects which resulted in controversial conclusions.[27]

So NIDA seemed to be content, in the seventies, with adopting an attitude of benign neglect with respect to cocaine. While unwilling to support new studies aimed at researching its damaging effects, they could not find in past medical literature sufficient scientific proof to justify the formulation of a strong indictment of cocaine similar to that expressed so clearly by Lewin or Hans Maier. But NIDA published research monographs at regular intervals to keep medical scientists and its grantees abreast of the latest developments in the field of drug dependence. NIDA's first publication on cocaine, printed in 1974, was a list of references including the book by Hans Maier, which was only listed in its French translation (*La Cocaïne*), along with 1800 other references, such as *The Gourmet*

Coke Book and articles from scientific journals and the lay press.[28] While some of Freud's contributions are listed (in their English translations or adaptations), the classic review by Lewin is not mentioned; neither are the basic contributions of Magnan, Guillain, Stein, Schnyder, Falke, and Bravetta and Invernizi, nor many other French, German, and Italian authors. The usefulness of the NIDA bibliography was very limited since the listings were in alphabetic order and not broken down into categories such as "chemistry," "toxicology," "pharmacology," or "clinical." However it contained statistics listing the number of publications on "psycho-social, socio-legal, ethnocultural, behavioral-animal" studies. In brief, it was a hodge-podge of little value to the researcher who might be looking for examples of the toxic effects of cocaine on man.

The next NIDA publication on cocaine, printed in 1975, listed sixty–nine articles and books abstracted from the scientific and popular literature on the "psychosocial aspects of human use of cocaine."[29] Four papers by Freud are listed, and he is also quoted eleven times in other analyses. Books by Mortimer, Crowley, Ashley, and the anonymous *Gourmet Coke Book* extolling the merits of cocaine and its lack of toxic effects are abstracted without comment. Maier and Lewin are not mentioned. Of the hundreds of clinical reports describing the damaging effects of the drug, only the one written by the Indian psychiatrist Bose is abstracted. The 1976 annotated bibliography prefigured the contention made in a subsequent (1977) NIDA publication which stated that "very little was known about cocaine with any certainty."[30]

NIDA, in the words of Dr. Robert Dupont, its director at that time, "awarded a million dollars each year between 1972 and 1976 to conduct research using modern pharmacological techniques and to support 40 research projects exploring aspects of cocaine from the chemistry of the substance to the characteristics of the users." In the foreword of the 1977 monograph on cocaine, Dr. Dupont says, "We are still to a large extent ignorant of the potential health hazards posed by this fascinating substance even though it was used by about two million Americans in the past year (1976)."[31] "And, yet," adds Dr. Dupont, "we know that cocaine can kill, and death occurs even when the drug is snorted rather than injected; we also know that cocaine is among the most powerfully reinforcing of all abused drugs, although not physically addictive." The monograph *Cocaine 1977* represents a sort of balancing act performed by NIDA's sponsored scientists between "what was known and not known about cocaine" and its implications for health. It was intended, according to Dr. Dupont, to become "a useful document for those interested in applying modern scientific knowledge to the serious social policy questions associated with cocaine use in America." Dr. Robert Peterson and Dr. Richard Stillman, the authors of *Cocaine 1977,* insist that their goal is

> to develop a picture of our current knowledge with special attention to its limitations. The authors have not tried to gloss over the areas of ignorance that exist nor to substitute unsubstantiated opinion for authoritative data. It is our belief that the needs of all readers are better served by as objective an assessment as is now possible rather than by more dogmatic assertions.[32]

Such statements indicate that their authors had dismissed the clinical reports of Lewin and Maier, who had demonstrated that cocaine, either sniffed or injected, is profoundly addictive, with most damaging effects on mind and body, and that its use spreads according to an epidemic mode when the drug is not strictly controlled.

Casual dismissal of these same early reports on cocaine is displayed in the paper written by the NIDA grantees Dr. Robert Byck and Craig Van Dyke, professors of psychiatry at Yale University, entitled "What are the Effects of Cocaine on Man?"[33] According to Byck and Van Dyke, the "*known*" effects of cocaine must be limited to those observed in a "controlled experimental situation, in a number of independent laboratories" similar to their own; and these known effects included only the following ones: local anesthesia, euphoria, and increases in blood pressure and heart rate. Sudden death by respiratory or cardiac arrest and convulsions, which may not readily be observed in a controlled laboratory situation, were considered by Byck and Van Dyke to be "anecdotal accounts" and were not mentioned by the authors, who concluded that "most of the effects of cocaine that seemed to be known are open to question." Their bibliography, consisting of twenty-four titles, lists only three European authors: Freud, Koller, and Aschenbrandt cited earlier in this book and who describe the positive properties of the drug. In any event, the conclusions of Byck and Van Dyke appeared to have been shared by the NIDA leadership which awarded the Yale psychiatrists, between 1974 and 1980, one million dollars to study the "acute effects of cocaine on man" and "cocaine effects and modification of euphoria in man."[34]

Some of the complications of cocaine use referred to as anecdotal by Byck and Van Dyke were, however, reported in *Cocaine 1977* by Dr. Ronald Siegel, a Los Angeles psychologist. He notes in his paper, "Cocaine: Recreational Use and Intoxication,"[35] that after heavy consumption, his patients, who are social recreational users of the drug, present "pseudo-hallucinations." However, Siegel claims these symptoms are different from the true hallucinations associated with incipient psychosis, and that the "cocaine bugs" described by Magnan in the last century are in reality little more than "itching sensations." Indeed, all of these adverse effects disappear when cocaine use becomes less intensified, as the user shifts to "more recreational regimes. In this sense users are capable of titrating their doses so as to circumvent adverse reactions." Siegel does not compare his observations with those of Hans Maier and refers to Lewin, not to express a dissenting view, but to quote the German pharmacologist's anecdote of a monkey addicted to cocaine.[36]

In the same monograph, another paper by two psychiatrists, Dr. Donald Wesson and Dr. David Smith, describes in more sobering terms the recreational use of cocaine among patients of Haight-Ashbury Free Medical Clinic of San Francisco.[37] The cases reported by Wesson and Smith indicate that cocaine will, especially when injected intravenously, produce hallucinations as well as psychosis and also severe depression during withdrawal. The authors' conclusion? "Cocaine is a drug of moderately high abuse potential," at the very least an ambiguous classification which is matched by their remarking, "Although most cocaine use, even in a social recreational setting does not produce adverse medical or psychological consequences, one should not necessarily conclude that cocaine is harmless." We are far from the blanket rejection of cocaine except for medical purposes that was articulated by Lewin and Maier. Psychiatrists Wesson and Smith are much closer to the stand that was, belatedly, taken by Freud who viewed moderate use of the drug as innocuous, but thought it could induce addiction and some toxic effects in susceptible persons. Many of the psychiatrists who have studied drug dependence hold similar, ambiguous views on cocaine's properties; their writings and pronouncements are characterized by a typical combination of claims for causality followed by denials of causality. They feel constrained to give a causal explanation but refuse to make definitive statements which could be later criticized for factual omissions. *Cocaine 1977* ends with a sobering analysis of the one hundred and eleven cocaine-related deaths reported by U.S. coroners between 1971 and 1976, indicating a more than twenty-fold increase in yearly incidence, from 2 to 58 within five years.[38]

Even these statistics were not alarming enough to justify a warning from NIDA to the American public of an impending major epidemic of cocaine use, a drug which had been branded, following the first epidemic at the turn of the century, as the most addictive and destructive of all drugs known to man. If one looks for a common thread to relate all of the statements which underestimate the social and health dangers of cocaine, from *Uber Coca* to the 1977 NIDA report, one finds that it has been spun by a few articulate and popular psychiatrists, who are frequently mentioned in these pages.

NIDA had taken a similarly timorous stand on marijuana during the preceding decade when the recreational use of the "harmless weed," fanned by the student revolt and the advocates of NORML, was sweeping the country. At that time, according to NIDA experts, there was only "anecdotal" evidence of the damaging effects of marijuana on the mental or physical health of users. For years, in my laboratory under controlled laboratory conditions, I studied the subtle damage induced by marijuana on cells of the immune system and reproductive organs. I organized international symposia on marijuana and wrote many articles and some scientific texts.[39] The response of NIDA to this research has been disappointing. Our grant applications were turned down or not renewed, a plight shared with other scientists who reported results indicating the damaging effects of marijuana.[40]

On the positive side, I found unexpected supporters, first from the American Council on Marijuana and Drug Education,[41] a group of public-spirited prominent citizens led by Marion and Olivia Gilliam, who sounded the alarm in the early seventies on the major dangers of illicit drug use for the future of America. A few years later I was to find supporters among the newly-formed parents' groups, PRIDE (Parents, Resource Institute for Drug Education)[42] and N.F.P. (National Federation of Parents for a Drug Free Youth).[43]

In the late seventies, while the use of marijuana and other addictive drugs was escalating and seemed to permeate American society, a grassroots movement of concerned and vocal parents appeared on the national scene. The adherents of this movement became my staunchest supporters. First from the traditional South and the solid mid-West, and then from all over the country, parents observed with dismay the damaging effects of marijuana smoking and illicit drug use on children, disrupting family life and impairing school performance. These first-hand observations could be made without the benefit of modern medical science which has no method to measure the impairing effects of marijuana intoxication on adolescent brain and behavior.

I joined the parents' movement as a father of three drug-free children and also as a scientist who had finally found a receptive audience to spread the message of the health hazards of marijuana and cocaine. Parents' groups took the lead in their communities and local schools to propound their simple message. *"No use of illicit drugs. No illegal use of licit drugs."* They put pressure on their elected representatives and supported legislation aimed at closing "paraphernalia" shops. The parents' groups received the dedicated support of the First Lady, Nancy Reagan; their political influence was strong enough to stop the implementation of marijuana "decriminalization," no small achievement. I found myself, for the first time, surrounded by committed allies. Among them are Dr. Thomas Gleaton and Dr. Keith Schuchard, professors at Georgia State University and co-founders of "PRIDE," which has become the largest and most effective organization for the prevention of drug dependence in the nation and the world. I also met Otto and Connie Moulton, a most dedicated couple from New England. They have committed their lives and resources to fighting the drug culture. Through their "Committees of Correspondence"[44] they inform the people of America on the health and social hazards of illicit drug consumption, which NIDA experts and many academics have been unwilling to spell out clearly.

I frequently exchanged phone calls with Gleaton or Moulton in order to keep abreast of the developments on the "drug front." In early 1980 they both expressed their concern about the rising use of cocaine among young people and also voiced their dismay about their difficulties in obtaining from NIDA a clear indictment of cocaine as a truly addictive drug. I looked up old observations of Lewin and Maier and after comparing them with the newer information collected in America in the sixties and seventies I wrote the following statement on October 28, 1980:

Cocaine: The Great Addicter

Cocaine is a chemical extracted from the leaf of the coca bush, a South American shrub. It is a white crystalline powder soluble in water.

It is used in medicine in highly diluted form as a local surface anesthetic agent applied to the mucous membranes of the nose and throat.

When absorbed in the blood stream by sniffing or snorting, it is a very potent drug: A tiny amount (1–3 milligrams) produces profound stimulating effects on the brain by releasing a chemical, norepinephrine, from the nerve endings.

It provokes a considerable mood elevation marked by a surge of excitement and a sense of expanded mental and physical power. Fatigue disappears, and mental acuity seems enhanced. These psychological effects are associated with an increase in heart rate, blood pressure, and breathing rate, and a decreased appetite.

This state of excitation and euphoria is followed within 30–60 minutes by a physical and psychological "let down feeling." Depression and dullness succeed to alertness; tenseness and edginess follow euphoria.

Lethal overdose of cocaine either snorted or injected has been regularly reported and is on the increase. Death is caused by heart failure or respiratory paralysis; convulsions also occur.

Chronic effect: The frequent snorting of cocaine produces burns and sores of the membranes which line the interior of the nose. Ear and nose specialists see more and more frequently, in chronic cocaine users, perforations of the septum, the cartilage separating the nostrils.

Physical symptoms of heavy cocaine use include cold sweats, pallor, uncontrolled tremors, heaviness of the limbs, aggressive behavior, insomnia, and weight loss.

Psychological symptoms are characterized by intense anxiety, depression and confusion, hallucinations (especially formication, the conviction that ants are crawling under one's skin) and paranoid delusions. These latter symptoms often require hospitalization in a psychiatric ward.

Rapid and marked tolerance develops to cocaine use (necessity to increase the dosage in order to obtain the initial effect).

Cocaine is the only drug, with amphetamines, which animals will self-administer until they die. This self-administration is the best example of the behavioral dependence created by cocaine which has been called the great addicter because of the profound craving that it creates in the brain of the user.

All of these damaging effects of cocaine in man, and their resulting destructive influences in Western society, were first observed one hundred years ago. They led to the establishment of strict legal national and international controls in order to limit the use of this drug to medical applications only. For fifty years, from 1910 to 1960, such regulations, coupled with social disapproval, were sufficient to curtail cocaine abuse to all but a very small group of high class society.

With the advent of the permissive, affluent society of the sixties, cocaine has known a new rush of popularity, especially in the U.S.

Today cocaine, at over $2,000 an ounce (3 times the price of gold), has become the champagne of drugs, the high class high, a status symbol of the rock star, the movie queen, the best selling author. It may also be found in the executive suite, the suburban living room for the cocktail hour, the college dorm and the high school locker.

The huge potential for profit explains the blossoming cocaine trade (mostly from Colombia). Furthermore, a lot of the cocaine is cut, short weighed and contains a number of adulterants. No more than 25% of the cocaine sold illicitly is pure. The rest is cut with innocuous substances such as sugars (mannitol, sucrose) or cheaper drugs such as procaine, lidocaine, benzocaine, and more dangerous ones such as amphetamines or quinine. These two last drugs may produce dangerous side effects. In spite of all, there are many buyers who happily pay $100 a gram for the pleasure of a cocaine fix.

If current estimates are accurate, at least 8 million Americans in the past year have sniffed cocaine or injected it into their blood stream.

In 1979, 15% of all American high school seniors had snorted cocaine at least once.

Ten years ago [1970], during one 12 month period, federal narcotics agents confiscated 25 pounds of cocaine. Last year [1979], over one ton was confiscated.

Head shops that once sold only marijuana paraphernalia now stock a full display of cocaine accessories (cheaper if bought by the dozen).

By far the most dangerous form of absorption of cocaine is by smoking the free base. This produces an intense rush, with rapid development of severe psychological and psychiatric symptoms requiring hospitalization.

Summing up: The use of cocaine in a society is a sign of its confusion and decline; it is the door open to self-destruction. It is high time that social taboos be restored against the great addicter.

PRIDE, the Committees of Correspondence, and the National Federation of Parents distributed tens of thousands of these pamphlets in schools across the nation, while Professor Sidney Cohen from the University of California at Los Angeles wrote a more extensive indictment of cocaine which was widely distributed by the American Council for Drug Education.[45] But how could we compete with the billions of messages tolerant of "recreational" cocaine use and which had been disseminated by the mass media for a decade and were still so often heard in a less strident but more subtle fashion? Our efforts to convince people of the devastating effects of cocaine were like those of the little Dutch boy attempting to prevent a major flood by putting his finger into a hole in the dike.

And so in the eighties I was drawn into a new battle against the further trivialization of cocaine use. This fight had to be waged by recalling the destructive properties of cocaine, scientifically documented but forgotten, and also by studying in the laboratory the mechanisms of its damaging effect. Foremost, we had to start rebuilding, from American grass roots, the cultural and ethical safeguards patiently erected by the outstanding reformers of America to control cocaine use, and which now lay in shambles. Upon this wreckage the new cocaine epidemic was spreading like wildfire all over the Americas, as I was to discover in the years ahead.

15

From Icy Norway to California Snow, 1982

Nowhere in America was the popularity of cocaine greater than in that paradise of earthly pleasures, California. A well-known TV personality on a nationwide show aptly remarked: "When it snows in California, everyone rushes outside to sniff his driveway." Cocaine use was to become increasingly prevalent among the well-heeled crowds of film and media in Los Angeles.

Over the airwaves rock lyrics extolled escaping on the stimulating wings of the champagne of drugs, cocaine. Eric Clapton's song was a top hit.

> When the day is done
> And you want to run
> Cocaine!
>
> When you've got bad news
> And you want to kick the blues
> Cocaine![1]

Dozens of pop lyrics thrilled millions with the excitement of coke and enticed untold numbers into trying it. Rock stars, and the best known among them, publicly flaunted their cocaine habit in full view of an amused and tolerant public. Already in 1975, Nicholas Von Hoffman,[2] in an article entitled "The Cocaine Culture, New Wave for the Rich and Hip," quotes a Los Angeles record producer, "There are certain clubs in this town where you feel out of place if you aren't wired to the teeth. That fast cocaine tempo!" and he adds, "It has come home to you that you can buy anything and do anything and you have to do it. How do you solve your problem? You get into cocaine."

Following the success of *Easy Rider* and *Superfly* in the early seventies, cocaine kept on appearing regularly on the screen. In the movie *Annie Hall*, Woody Allen is offered a snort of a most expensive white powder. Impressed, he takes a closer look at the gem-studded gold pill-box, sneezes, and the cocaine is blown over the carpet! In *Hannah and her Sisters* one of the sisters snorts cocaine as casually as some smoke a cigarette.

The film *Atlantic City* describes the odyssey of a pound of cocaine from dealer to dealer, gradually decreasing in strength and increasing in price. The multiple transactions cause the death of the traffickers, except for the hero of this macabre adventure, masterfully played by Burt Lancaster.

Another movie, *Scarface,* on the life of the gangster, Al Capone, depicts a grand game of cocaine traffic where dealers get power, money, and beautiful women — while rival gangs gun each other down.

The media mirror and exaggerate at the same time current social trends and, by focusing on drugs, encourage their social acceptance, while glamorizing the latent fantasies of viewers.

The trivialization of cocaine use, so manifest in the media and on the screen, was also apparent in the reports of ever-increasing inflows of the drug, little counteracted by frequent seizures of drug shipments by law enforcement officials. Fleets of planes flew in their daily cargo of white gold, first extracted from coca leaves in Peru or Bolivia and then refined in Colombia. Distribution routes, controlled by the powerful and murderous Colombian mafia, kept the whole country supplied from the east coast to California. The new method of "body packing" was used to smuggle cocaine from South America to the United States and Europe. The "body packer," or mule, will ingest cocaine–filled packets along with a constipating agent.[3] After passage through customs, the packer expels the packets and the contents are recovered. As many as 100 such packs containing 5 to 10 grams of cocaine each have been transported by a single person in this fashion. In some instances, the packet will burst open and the bearer will be severely intoxicated. As a result he may die of cocaine overdose. This mode of transport has led to the systematic X-ray of suspicious–looking travelers coming from South America. But mostly cocaine arrived in shipments of hundreds of pounds

The Drug Enforcement Agency announced the seizure of *tons* of cocaine while admitting that the catch represented no more than a fraction, ten percent at most, of the amount consumed. And more cocaine (2.5 tons) was seized in the first half of 1982 than in the entire year of 1981 (2 tons). On the basis of the seizure of 2.5 tons of cocaine over a six-month period, it was estimated that 14 tons of cocaine would be consumed in 1982 in the United States, providing enough of the drug to supply several million users.[4] Surveys performed in New York State alone indicated that from 1975 to 1981 those who had used cocaine increased from 94,000 to 252,000, and those who had used cocaine in the month of the interview rose from 6,000 to 29,000.[5] All social classes and age groups were involved, with a "higher incidence of use among youth" reported by the annual national surveys of Johnston and collaborators.[6] Paradoxically, the experts Edgar Adams and Jack Durrell[7] of the National Institute on Drug Abuse found that there was an apparent leveling off in overall national prevalence of cocaine use when they made two major surveys for the Institute between 1979 and 1982.

The dreaded effects of the trivialization of cocaine use in California became widely known in the Spring of 1982. One of the most popular of screen and TV stars, John Belushi, was found dead after being injected by a woman companion with a mixture of cocaine and heroin. This practice, known as "speed balling," is the only way, according to experienced drug users, to reach a climax of pleasure within instants. Shortly before this episode, Paul Newman's son died of drug overdose as did hundreds of youths across the land. In 1982 in California cocaine became a bigger killer than heroin.

The media thrived on the sensationalism of these events and gave top billing to disheartening reports on the gradual rise of cocaine use in all social groups, from the high school student to the professor, from foreman to boss, from teller to bank manager, and from actor to athlete.

As cocaine addiction spread, a new, more destructive, mode of absorption by smoking the "free base" became popular. Free base is made by dissolving the cocaine powder in water, adding a strong alkali, and extracting the base with a volatile, flammable solvent like ether, a substance which may easily catch fire. Richard Pryor, a famous entertainer, suffered very severe burns in 1982 while preparing his free base. This dangerous and expensive process was replaced a few years later by a much simpler and cheaper one used for the fabrication of another form of cocaine base—"crack." To make crack, the cocaine hydrochloride is dissolved in alkaline water, bicarbonate is added, the water is evaporated by boiling, and the crackling whitish residue is ready for smoking. Either form of smoked free base cocaine is rapidly absorbed through the lungs into the bloodstream, and reaches very high brain concentrations, evoking an intense rush and a compulsive desire to continue smoking. As a result the toxic effects of cocaine appear rapidly and are identical to those described following intravenous use, or those observed in the coca paste smokers of Peru by Raoul Jeri:[8] marked weight loss, severe insomnia, manic depression or paranoid psychosis with hallucinations, serious lung complications, convulsions, and respiratory or cardiac arrest.

During all this time drug experts, sponsored by NIDA, were continuing their studies on the effects of cocaine which, in the words of the new director of NIDA, Dr. William Pollin, "had become the drug of greatest national concern from a public health point of view and of particularly high interest from the research and scientific point of view."[9] A new conference of cocaine experts was called by NIDA in 1982 at a time when the experts of the Institute were still uncertain as to the progression of the epidemic and were awaiting, according to Pollin, "further clarification of the exact nature of current trends in prevalence of cocaine use."[10] One of the major rediscoveries made by the scientific experts of NIDA was reported at that 1982 conference by Dr. Reese Jones who stated that "a true withdrawal syndrome following cocaine use seems compelling."[11] He mentions depression, social withdrawal, tremor, muscle pain, eating disturbances, and changes in sleep patterns. "For many patients," adds Jones, "it appears that the withdrawal symptoms make discontinuing cocaine impossible so long as the drug is available."

The same observations were made by Lewin a century before but were considered anecdotal, as were the more recent ones by Maier and his colleagues, who, in addition, did not hesitate to voice a strong condemnation of the recreational use of the drug. Such a critical stand was a difficult one for NIDA to take in view of the social acceptance of cocaine which was reported by Dr. Ronald Siegel at that same 1982 conference. He claimed that many social users of cocaine are capable of controlling use with no escalation to larger toxic doses.[12] Professor Herbert Kleber and Frank Gawin of Yale University, who had been exerting great efforts in researching new treatments for cocaine dependency, reported their latest findings in the *Proceedings* of the same 1982 NIDA Cocaine Conference.[13] By their own admission the results obtained were quite disappointing, regardless of the treatment, which included group or individual psychotherapy associated with the latest medications for hospitalized and ambulatory patients. They concluded "that single focus approaches are generally ineffective in the treatment of cocaine addiction and that more research was required." Such recommendations contrasted with those formulated by Maier fifty years earlier: "The only attitude that the physician must adopt when confronted with cocaine use of any type is to absolutely forbid the patient to use the drug."

The American psychiatric establishment in 1982 was not ready to adopt such a radical stand which Freud would have disapproved and which NIDA was in no position to endorse in a country where social acceptance of cocaine use was becoming entrenched. So NIDA could be said to have been compelled to take a wait-and-see attitude, which it had adopted since its inception. NIDA was content to hold a cocaine conference every three or four years to find out what had happened in the field as the epidemic progressed. In May of 1982, the National Council on Marijuana and Drug Education, which had always taken a firm stand against the recreational use of drugs, decided to hold another National Conference on Cocaine, this time in Santa Monica, California. The California location had been purposefully selected and the declared objective was to determine "the risk to the users of this drug particularly in its free base form."

I was invited to the conference by its convener, Dr. Robert Dupont, former head of the National Institute on Drug Abuse and new president of the American Council on Marijuana and Drug Education. The day before the California meeting opened I was to speak at a colloquium in Norway on the use of illicit drugs. So on a Spring morning my plane landed in the chilly mists of Oslo airport still in the grips of its long winter.

I was greeted by Dr. Harold Benestadt and two of his university colleagues who had invited me to give the keynote speech at the National Meeting of the Norwegian Student Association whose theme was: "Drugs in the Year 2000."

"Thank you for coming to Norway, even for a few hours," said Benestadt. "We have a serious problem in this country. We expect you to speak on the dangers of cannabis use and of the escalation to cocaine."

We barely made it to the plenary session.

The large conference room of the Hotel Scandinavia, resplendent with its crystal chandeliers, was packed. Physicians, educators, social workers, and students browsed through the folders of materials handed out by smiling hostesses, or adjusted their headphones for a simultaneous translation of my speech. On the stage I joined a dozen participants seated at a long table covered with green felt. At ten o'clock sharp, the Minister of Justice, Mona Rokke, a tall slender young man, opened the meeting.

"Until recently," he said, "drugs were unknown to Norwegians — except for alcohol, of course. However, alcoholism only touched a small portion of our population which had one of the lowest rates of alcohol consumption per capita in the world. In the last few years, in spite of rationing and high prices, alcohol use has been on the rise. At the same time, illicit toxic substances have appeared on the market — first hashish, then hallucinogenic substances, followed by L.S.D. and heroin, and today cocaine."

I looked at the audience, which was no different from the ones I had addressed in France and in the United States. Next to adults, parents, and educators I recognized students, attentive and eager to be briefed on the latest scientific developments in the field.

Applause broke out after the minister's closing plea to join forces and "halt the spread of a plague of modern times which threatens the future of our youth and of our country." The words had a familiar ring. I then took the stand to speak on the topic requested by the organizers, "The Medical Dangers of Hashish and Cocaine." I illustrated my talk with slides and the film on the self-administration of cocaine by a monkey. After my presentations, I received questions from the floor.

"If these drugs are so harmful to our health, why do so many people use them?" inquired a young Viking with a curly blond beard.

I had been asked that question before. It seemed logical to assume that modern science had the means to find out why people use drugs. Once the causes of drug-taking were determined, prevention measures and treatment methods could then be rationally defined. My answer was simple:

"Because drugs trigger pleasure in the user's brain." I nearly added: "Why does one make love?"

"But pleasure should not be a fault, a sin," replied the student, expressing the prevailing philosophy of his time.

"No, only when it leads to suffering and degradation." This value judgment did not seem to satisfy the student. I added, "I will also give another answer to your first question about drug consumption. Drugs are increasingly consumed once they become readily available and socially acceptable, regardless of prevalent political or social conditions: unemployment or prosperity, a democratic or an authoritarian regime."

I would have liked to pursue this conversation, which is at the center of drug policy prevention, but the chair thanked me and gave the floor to the next speaker. I slipped away to catch my plane for the States.

After a ten-hour flight, three of them at the Concorde's supersonic speed, and thanks to the time differential, I reached the sunlit shores of the Pacific on the same evening. During that unending journey into daylight, I had time to reflect on the Norwegian student's question. Why do so many young people from Western nations use drugs nowadays, and especially the privileged youth favored by health, intelligence, and affluence? Why this rage to escape into a dream induced by mind-bending substances once shunned by their forebears?

How could the scientist be expected to resolve a human problem when he lacked methods to measure all of the variables involved? While scientists have the ability to unravel some of the secrets of nature, they lack the power to fathom the meaning of life and the prospect of human destiny that are threatened by drug addiction. Furthermore, by its very nature, it is doubtful that scientific inquiry is capable of finding solutions to existential human problems concerning life, death, love, or the future of man. The scientist is no more endowed by supernatural power than any other person.

I doubted that the California Conference on Cocaine, opening the next day, would offer answers to these weighty questions, but at least I was going to have the opportunity to meet the new American experts on cocaine.

16

An Academic Confrontation on Cocaine

The California Conference on Cocaine met near Santa Monica
in a splendid oceanside hotel surrounded by gardens with palm
trees and glowing hibiscus and where one could hear the inter-
mittent sounds of the ocean breakers unfurling on the long,
sunny beach just beyond Pacific Boulevard.

Several hundred participants gathered in the conference
room: psychologists, psychiatrists, and social workers eager to
help their patients addicted to cocaine but not knowing quite
how to proceed. They reminded me of Good Samaritans, ready
to assist the unfortunate ones knocking at the door for help.
However, the afflicted of the 20th century are well-fed and
well-housed, and suffer from so deep an ailment that charity
alone cannot rescue them. They are captive to a poison of the
brain which they cannot give up and which destroys their lives.

The main speakers at the colloquium were, in addition to
the California drug specialists, Sidney Cohen, Ronald Siegel,
and David Smith — all three psychiatrists; and two out of town
guests, Dr. Raoul Jeri from Peru and myself.

Dr. Sidney Cohen,[1] the recognized American dean of
drug experts, opened the meeting with an historical survey of
cocaine use. As a psychiatrist, he was aware of the controversy
that had pitted Freud against Lewin a century ago and he
compared that distant period with our own.

His presentation drew few questions. After all, in this age
of electronics and artificial hearts, why dwell on ancient history?

Dr. Ronald Siegel[2] took the podium next and was greeted
with warm applause. Siegel, a young psychologist, professor of
psychiatry at the University of California Los Angeles, spoke

with a confidence acquired in the course of frequent media appearances as a drug expert.

Tall, slender, peering through horn-rimmed glasses, a half-smile on his lips, he promptly put his audience at ease with the anecdotal account of screen and public life celebrities whom he would not name but who were said to gather and snort the white powder with zest after attending a benefit gala for the victims of drug abuse. He next reported his observations on a group of one hundred cocaine users he had studied in Los Angeles from 1970 to 1982. They were young, between the ages of eighteen and thirty, and mainly students, with a sprinkling of professionals and other adults: doctors, lawyers, writers, teachers, secretaries, and housewives. They initially snorted one to four grams of powder a month. Before trying cocaine they had consumed alcohol and smoked pot. They started on coke at parties, to "follow the crowd" and keep up with their peers, moved by a curiosity about a substance that supposedly stimulated minds and hearts.

"The rediscovery of cocaine in the seventies was unavoidable," declared Siegel, "because its stimulating and pleasure-causing properties reinforce the American character, with its initiative, its energy, its restless activity, and its boundless optimism." After ten years, from 1980 on, Dr. Siegel had lost touch with nearly half of his patients. About ten of them, he said, gave up the habit; one–fourth remained moderate users without seriously damaging their health; and one–fourth had become excessive users, smoking cocaine free base with, as a result, damaging physical and psychological effects. The free-basers tried to treat their dependency by observing periods of abstinence and resorting to substitute drugs, such as amphetamines, or local anesthetics, like novocaine.

Siegel concluded that many cocaine users are perfectly capable of controlling their consumption and avoiding the escalation to compulsive use. Others fail and run the risk of suffering from toxic accidents. His closing words, greeted with loud applause, pleased everyone.

The participants who had paid a hundred dollars each to attend the conference were especially anxious to hear about the treatment recommended by Dr. Siegel for "non-recreational" addiction. Siegel favored out-patient treatment over confinement in an institution. Indeed, he claimed, cocaine addicts will eventually have to abstain from the drug in an environment where it is, and where it will remain for the foreseeable future, readily available; they must therefore be treated in such a milieu. "You can't treat a fish out of water," he said.

"Could you explain more specifically what your method is?" asked a young lady, a spokesperson for the Federation of Parents for Drug Free Youth.

"Well, to start, you've got to gradually decrease the daily intake of cocaine. The recreational users must learn how to ration themselves, and many do it without difficulty. Others resort to commercially available substances that simulate cocaine. I won't mention them; everyone here knows what they are. Another strategy is to abstain periodically from cocaine for several days or several months and allow the body to recuperate. All contact with the drug, its users, and its pushers must be avoided. Leaving for a vacation, reading reports on the harmful effects of the drug, or looking up some of the many drug-related news stories are good antidotes."

"You mean provide a negative reinforcement to counteract the positive reinforcement of cocaine?" asked a psychotherapist.

"Exactly," answered Siegel. "The best negative reinforcing strategy is called, 'contingency contracting.' An addict will sign a contract with his employer in which he asks to be penalized in case of a relapse into cocaine addiction. You see there are many strategies; each one must be well–timed and adapted for individual use under a therapist's guidance."

"Which are you recommending: individual or group therapy?"

"Well, it all depends on the subject. There are no general rules. I think that a group, with its dynamics and its shared experiences presents a definite advantage, especially for impulsive abusers. I'm personally involved in this kind of group therapy, with three or four sessions a week, and I find it to be very effective, but we can talk about that later this afternoon."

After Dr. Siegel's presentation, I took the floor to discuss, with the help of slides, the pharmacological properties of cocaine: how it modifies brain function by stimulating the production of chemical substances related to adrenalin, a process which explains the excitement generated by the drug. These biochemical changes occur in the same nervous pathways which induce pleasure and reward, and have been pro-grammed by nature to favor activities related to survival of the individual and the species: search for food and reproduction. In the long run, cocaine use so profoundly alters brain chemistry that it leads to paranoia and insanity.

I described experiments on the self-administration of cocaine in human volunteers. When given the opportunity, men, just like monkeys, choose an injection of cocaine over that of a salt solution and keep increasing the dose. The ensuing tolerance translates into a need for increasingly large quantities to maintain the initial euphoria. I insisted on the misleading distinction between "physical" and "psychological" dependence of addictive drugs.[3] "Physical dependence" in reality only describes the symptoms specific to the withdrawal symptoms from opiates which are manifested by disabling but not life-threatening clinical signs such as pain, anxiety, fever, digestive troubles, trembling, and nausea. By contrast the quiet urge leading an opiate addict to consume heroin, even when he has no longer any withdrawal symptoms, had been defined as "psychic addiction."

This distinction which spans most of the recent psychiatric literature on drugs has led many to believe that the opiates and heroin were the only truly addictive drugs. As a result, it has been claimed that cocaine, cannabis, or tobacco were not addictive because cessation of their use is not accompanied by a full-blown withdrawal symptom of the opiate type. According to these opinions the use of cocaine may be readily interrupted if the user exerted enough "will power." And yet cocaine use results in an addiction which is as compelling as that induced by heroin, a fact noted by Lewin and Maier at the turn of the century, and only recently rediscovered. Cocaine induces biochemical changes in the brain, which are physical in nature and which linger on; the cessation of cocaine use is also characterized by withdrawal symptoms, different from those of opiate addiction and characterized by depression and marked disturbances of sleep patterns manifested by abnormal brain wave patterns.

The clear-cut distinction between psychic and physical dependence illustrates the old dichotomy between mind and body, a belief perpetuated by Freud who thought that certain patterns of behavior were "all in the mind." Modern neurophysiology and psychopharmacology no longer justify this concept of complete separation of mind and body since soma and psyche are inextricably interwoven.

I also proposed a new classification of dependence-producing drugs according to their common properties, which distinguish them from therapeutic drugs. Impairment of the transmission of nerve signals by addictive drugs through the brain (neurotransmission) will alter all of its functions, feeling capacity, intellectual ability, and memory. Such a global impairment of brain function will manifest itself through acute and chronic symptoms. Two acute manifestations will appear after every intake of an addictive drug, and are caused by reversible impairment of neurotransmission. They are a feeling of pleasure and reward, and a blurring of intellectual functions which prevent an authentic relationship between brain and environment. These two acute symptoms of the drug experience are associated with three more lasting ones which are typical of chronic addiction: tolerance, abstinence, and reinforcement. Tolerance develops after repeated ingestion of the addictive drug, and is a state which requires an increasing dose in order to obtain the initial effect. The abstinence syndrome, or withdrawal, follows the interruption of regular drug use, and is manifest by unpleasant, painful, depressive manifestations. Tolerance and abstinence are caused by a chronic impairment of brain function, which at times becomes irreversible. And last the symptom of addiction is called "reinforcement," the property of the drug which leads the addict to repeated self-administration. This reinforcing property is related to the predominant memory induced by the drug experience, and which is printed into the brain. The reinforcing property of addictive drugs is the basis for the drug-seeking and drug-consuming behavior which is so deeply ingrained that it may reappear even after a long period of abstinence.

To conclude, I ran Dr. Seevers' film once more which I called "Always More" and which shows a monkey who self-administers cocaine by pressing furiously on a lever, until he goes into convulsions.

My presentations received scant applause.

One person asked if the film and slides were available to the public. Another suggested that these documents would be effective in prevention programs for high school students. But the biochemical alterations of the brain which explain the behavior of cocaine addicts seemed to have gone unnoticed by the audience.

Little did I suspect that I had just set the stage for the next speaker, Dr. Raoul Jeri,[4] professor of neurology at San Marcos University in Lima, Peru.

Dr. Jeri is a descendant both of the Indians of Peru and of their Spanish conquistadores. To this duel inheritance he owes certain physical features: a medium height, a slight build, an angular profile, and a dark complexion. The sad and thoughtful look he cast over the audience seemed to mirror the tragedy of human destiny.

In hesitant English and with the help of slides, Jeri described some of the damage wrought in South America by the epidemic use of cocaine paste which has been smoked since the early seventies. He reported the first cases in Lima in 1974, and many others were observed subsequently in all the large cities of Peru and those of neighboring Bolivia and Colombia.

Basic coca paste is the raw material from which cocaine is extracted. The coca leaves are soaked in a mixture of sulfuric acid, bicarbonate, and kerosene until they form a paste, which is dried in the sun. The paste contains fifty to sixty percent cocaine base which, unlike cocaine chlorhydrate, is not destroyed by the heat of a burning cigarette but is vaporized in the inhaled smoke. Currently thousands of coca paste smokers, *pastaleros* as they are called, mostly between the ages of twelve and twenty-five, have become irretrievably addicted to cocaine. All social groups are affected, from the unemployed to the affluent, from the blue-collar worker to the senior executive.

Pastaleros begin smoking tobacco and from there go on to marijuana joints which, before long, they mix with coca paste. The immediate effect on the smoker is an extraordinary feeling of bliss. Less than one hour after this indescribable pleasure the pastalero is plunged into deep anxiety and compelled to inhale another dose in order to rid himself of his anguish and retrieve his euphoria. Very soon he is caught in a pattern of compulsive behavior entirely directed towards the purchase and the consumption of the drug. He smokes dozens of cigarettes in succession until he drops with exhaustion and imperils his life. Within a few weeks he suffers from visual, tactile and auditory hallucinations, accurately described by Lewin a century ago;

and ultimately from acute dementia. The subject can experience severe paranoia and possibly commit murder or suicide.

Coca paste smokers, whatever their origin or their status in life, be they outstanding professionals, successful business executives, juvenile delinquents, or model schoolchildren, rapidly get hooked on a drug which becomes the center of their lives, as if they were the victims of a blind infatuation. Job, family, school, nothing counts: the same physical, intellectual, and moral deterioration awaits them all. Some die of convulsions, others of heart attacks.

Dr. Jeri summarized:

> Coca paste intoxication resembles a malignant disease featuring a gradual personality change which parallels the one observed in grave, incurable cases of dementia. *I would like to warn the U.S. against the plague which has reached its borders. I should also caution you that, not only does the recreational or experimental use of cocaine have no place in society, but that all pasta smokers abuse the substance. The trivialization of cocaine use is a curse on humanity.*

Ludwig Lewin, a hundred years ago, expressed himself in identical terms and so did Maier a little later, but, nowadays, in California, Freud's faulty theories on cocaine's lack of addictive potential seem to be winning more disciples among young physicians than are Lewin's or Maier's medical reports on the habit-forming property of this drug.

Dr. Jeri's closing remarks were followed by an uneasy silence, soon interrupted by the first question.

"How do you treat coca paste smokers?"

"We have found no medical treatment for cocaine addiction. All the methods used in Peru, be they in-patient detoxification, prolonged periods of confinement for rehabilitation, chemical treatments with tranquilizers, or lobotomies, are very disappointing. The relapse rate, whatever the treatment, is very high, between fifty and eighty percent."

"Did you say 'lobotomy'?" inquired someone.

"Yes, surgical lobotomy, 'cyngulotomy' to be precise, is performed in desperate cases on incurable repeaters, often upon request by the family and with the patient's consent."

"How barbaric," muttered my neighbor, probably voicing the general disapproval of such a procedure.

Dr. Jeri's presentation ended the morning session and had fascinated me. Proof had been given that one hundred years of unprecedented progress in the field of medical therapy had barely modified the course of cocaine addiction. The brain of Homo sapiens remained as vulnerable as ever to the temptation of cocaine and its addictive character.

The Conference participants gathered for lunch and I took a seat next to Ronald Siegel.

"Don't you think the high price of cocaine has limited its abuse?" I asked him.

"Not in the studies I presented this morning. As a matter of fact, fourteen of my subjects, occasional recreational users since 1974, have made careers in law, business, and medicine. Only three, one a physician, abused the drug when their income increased."

"But three out of fourteen — that represents over twenty percent of your sample," I retorted.

"Yes, but the majority still falls in the category of recreational users! So the notion that cocaine use is limited by its high price is not supported by the study I conducted between 1973 and 1982."

"Do you intend to follow the progress of these addicts beyond 1982?"

"Yes, if we receive enough funding from the government, we will."

Curious to know the price of the group therapy treatment briefly described by Professor Siegel in his presentation, I inquired about the frequency and the length of the sessions.

"Each session lasts ninety minutes and includes ten patients. The sessions meet four times a week and the treatment lasts a month."

"And how much does the treatment cost each patient?"

Siegel didn't seem to hear my question and I had to repeat it several times. Finally he answered me, lowering his voice as if he did not wish to be overheard: "One hundred and fifty dollars."

"Per week?"

"No, per session."

A quick mental calculation produced some figures: four sessions per week represent over $2400 per month and per patient. A therapist with ten patients could collect more than $24,000 in one month.

"And what was your reaction to Jeri's expose?"

"I believe, as he does, that smoking cocaine paste is dangerous. I repeat, smoking cocaine base."

"Do you mean to say that other forms of consumption are not as dangerous?"

"Exactly," replied Siegel. "I must add that stable recreational users know how to control their use of the substance and consume it knowingly. They believe that cocaine is an ideal drug, that it enhances their social lives; it's easy to carry around, effective within moments and for a foreseeable time, and with only few unpleasant after-effects."

I was reminded of Freud who took one hundred milligrams of cocaine before attending a dinner party at the home of the famous Professor Charcot in Paris; one hundred years later another psychiatrist was recognizing the redeeming effects of the drug on occasional consumers eager to improve their brilliance at social gatherings. The debate between Freud and Lewin had resumed but this time the psychiatrist seemed to be winning over the pharmacologist.

The afternoon session, devoted to the treatment of cocaine addiction, enjoyed an attentive audience. Dr. Siegel and Dr. David Smith, another leading therapist in drug addiction, shared the stage and waxed eloquent as they described the cases of cocaine addiction they had diagnosed and treated. All of their patients were strangely similar: regardless of their profession, sex, or age, they shared a passion for the drug, and the same unrelenting craving described by Lewin and Maier.[5]

Some patients, who came in a state of extreme agitation or deep anxiety, had to be treated with a tranquilizer like Valium which was injected intravenously in the course of the consultation. Unfortunately, this treatment yielded only temporary relief and could not be frequently repeated because tranquilizers are also addictive substances with unwanted side effects.

Other patients presenting symptoms of paranoia or dementia had to be hospitalized and treated with the same medications administered to schizophrenics. This treatment was effective to restore the addict to sanity but did not prevent him from relapsing after he had left the hospital.

All of these reports confirmed those of Lewin and Maier which had concluded that medical or psychiatric treatment of cocaine addiction was ineffective. Long-term rehabilitation in a drug-free environment was admittedly a possibility mentioned by Siegel and Smith, but in their opinion this solution could not be generalized and required the full consent of the addict. Staunchly opposed to any infringement on individual freedom and rejecting the coercive methods of totalitarian systems, they would occasionally recommend to consenting addicts an extended stay in a drug-free therapeutic community.

"However," commented Siegel, "there are few volunteers for this kind of treatment. It's costly because it requires a lengthy job interruption and a 'social dis-insertion,' followed by a 're-insertion' in an environment where drugs are available."

In brief, our expert therapists have little to offer the hard core cocaine addicts who suffer from a disease which has no other cure but total and permanent abstinence, a difficult option to advocate in the climate of tolerance towards drug use which prevails in California. These therapists will, of course, provide their patients with immediate relief in the form of kind words and tranquilizers. Such temporary measures follow an ago-old charitable tradition, with the difference that the starving poor of yester-year in need of room and board could be relieved more lastingly by bread and warmth alone. It would certainly be unfair to scorn today's Good Samaritans who are caring for cocaine addicts. Conforming to a drug-consuming society, they must help with ineffective measures the victims of a social deviance which they refuse to be the only ones to condemn. They are as much captives of their permissive social environment as the addicts are of cocaine.

In the course of the conference, the theses of Freud and Lewin had been, in fact, touched upon by both Siegel and Jeri. But, reversing a century-old stand, American intellectuals were today more inclined to listen to Dr. Siegel's interpretation than to Dr. Jeri's. I was convinced that the cost to society of such a choice would be staggering. I wondered, at the same time, why today's scholars casually ignore the lessons of past and present history.

17

Dr. Timothy Leary and the Media

The final exercises of the California Conference on cocaine assembled a star-studded panel of TV and movie moguls from Los Angeles. On the stage, high ranking executives of the major networks, CBS, NBC, and ABC, rubbed elbows with directors of the three largest Hollywood studios.

Each spokesman in turn took a strong stand against drugs, especially cocaine, pledging to fight its trivialization through enforcing a strict compliance with their code of ethics. This mutual admiration society, with its members on a first name basis — Bob, Jim, and Charlie — heaped praise on the fine standards upheld by their respective enterprises: The American film and television industry was one of the best in the world, it dominated the foreign market and could barely meet the clamor for its productions. While recognizing a few unfortunate slips here and there, all of the panelists declared themselves proud of their record. One of the speakers suggested that the best way to fight drug addiction was to treat drugs like tobacco: put them on the open market and eliminate the illegal traffic that breeds crime.

"Actually, the model is already in place in Great Britain."

The man's ignorance was disarming, matched only by the naïveté of his approving peers seated around him on the stage.

Are these affluent executives with their benevolent attitudes sincere, I wondered, or are they dupes of their subordinates? It is common knowledge that cocaine users are numerous in showbusiness. It is even rumored in Los Angeles that, in recent years, important sums are written into the production budget of films for the purchase of the white powder.

After hearing all this, I asked the gentlemen of the panel if they planned to take any measures to avoid filming actors smoking marijuana or snorting cocaine. A brief silence followed, finally broken by the president of a large TV network, a suave, quiet, and reassuring figure. In a slightly patronizing manner he ventured to say that in an age of electronic media and supersonic flights, the twentieth century American public had come of age and films merely reflected acceptable social practices. His neighbor approved, emphatically warning against censorship that had stifled the voices of an Oscar Wilde and a James Joyce, and more recently, during the McCarthy era, had persecuted some of the best script writers.

"The United States," he declared, "is the torch–bearer of liberty on our planet. Our mission is to preserve freedom, not to snuff it."

The audience applauded enthusiastically. All was for the best in the best of affluent worlds where millions of dollars worth of cocaine are sold, smoked, and snorted daily.

The panel broke up, and the main symposium participants gathered for a television interview to be aired on the major networks. The stage was set on Pacific Boulevard, under the noon sun, near a park ringed with palm trees, overlooking the expanse of Santa Monica Beach.

The star of the show was, unquestionably, Dr. Timothy Leary,[1] who made an uninvited appearance but was immediately spotted by the media. Great priest of the so–called "psychedelic" experiments which allow people to enhance their field of consciousness by consuming hallucinogenic drugs, Leary had known his hour of glory in the sixties. A disciple of Aldous Huxley,[2] who was the first advocate of drug induced mind-expanding practices, Leary went well beyond his mentor's ideas. Far from experimenting discreetly within a select circle of initiates, he widely proselytized the use of L.S.D. to "explore the subconscious." While a professor of psychology at Harvard, he had encouraged his students to embark on trips into the inner world of dreams and hallucinations. He exhorted millions of young people to "do drugs" and to follow the celebrated motto: "Turn on, tune in, drop out"—a call for youth to "get high," to "listen with a brain impaired by drugs," and finally "to become socially marginal." Hundreds of thousands of young Americans, enthusiastically following his appeal, entered the phantasmagoric universe created by drugs from which some never returned.

After Leary lost his job at Harvard in 1963, he joined the counter-culture. Sentenced to ten years in prison for drug use, he escaped from jail and fled to Algeria and then to Afghanistan where he was arrested. Extradited and reincarcerated in California, he was freed after five years. Thriving on the public's persistent nostalgia for the glamour and the wild dreams of the sixties, which he personified, he started a new career as author and lecturer.

Tall, slender, deeply tanned under a shock of white hair, his sport shirt open at the neck, Dr. Timothy Leary was the first target of questions from the Press.

"Tim," asked a reporter, "I heard you say that there are no dangerous drugs. Is that true?"

"Well, that's my way of looking at it. The real problem with drugs is the stupidity of most users. Intelligent people are going to use drugs intelligently. The brain is structured to present hundreds of points of entry or 'receptor sites.' Obviously these receptor sites have been created for a purpose: I believe that their function is to receive drugs. Therefore there are no dangerous drugs. Nevertheless, many people use drugs dangerously."

"Since, you've taken a stand on drugs in the past, can you tell us now what you think of cocaine?"

"Obviously, cocaine is the drug of the day. Isn't it the seventh largest business in the country? It's the drug of the 80's because this decade is facing the facts. We're in an age of realism and toughness."

"And why do you think cocaine is called the marijuana of the eighties?"

"Because it's well adapted to our times. Of course the "narcs" who are cracking down on its use rant and rave about the dangers of that miserable powder, which is, in reality, a harmless substance. Amphetamines are much more dangerous, not to mention alcohol, the most common and harmful of all drugs. I can't understand why some people are trying to make cocaine into a dreadful and evil plague, unless it's the traffickers from Peru who can use the publicity."

"How about yourself, Tim—what do you think of cocaine?"

"You mean as a user?"

"Yes."

"It's a drug that causes euphoria, quite pleasant and

sparkling like champagne. You feel powerful, as if you controlled the world — and intelligent, much more than you actually are. I've never turned down cocaine, except after midnight
if I want a good night's sleep."

"When you say 'a good night's sleep,' is that really why
you turn down cocaine?" laughed the reporter.

"Not always," chuckled Leary. "It depends on the company I'm keeping."

"If I can pick up on your hint, Tim, what do you think of
cocaine as an aphrodisiac?"

"It's a hard question to answer. Aphrodisiacs vary from
subject to subject but connoisseurs generally agree that L.S.D.
is the most aphrodisiac of all drugs [Dr. Leary who initiated his
students in L.S.D. when he taught at Harvard in the 60's had
some knowledge on the subject.] It's a fact that marijuana has
been used for over twenty-five hundred years by those who
wanted to improve their amorous performances. About every
week new drugs appear on the market, like "empathy," "XDC,"
all aphrodisiacs. So take your pick."

"Is it true more women than men favor cocaine?"

"All I've heard is that two snorts of cocaine put you in the
mood for love, but if the dose gets higher, then the mood
turns."

Leary laughed as he smoothed his silver locks which had
been blown by the ocean breeze. The journalist, who seemed to
be a connoisseur in matter of drugs, frowned:

"But Tim, why L.S.D.? Isn't it a drug that disrupts the
brain and doesn't do much to put a person in a romantic
mood?"

Leary shook his head.

"It depends on the individual. It's really all in the mind."

The journalist looked at me. "Your turn now," he said as
he introduced me to Leary: "You probably know Dr. Nahas."

"Yes, I've heard about him. Who doesn't know 'Marijuana Nahas'? But I've never had the pleasure of meeting him."

He extended a friendly hand.

"Hello, Gabe."

I made an effort to respond in as friendly a manner.

"Didn't you hear," I asked him, "what Dr. Jeri told us this
morning?"

"You've got to be completely nuts to smoke cocaine,"
agreed Leary. "I've always said it. Anyway, South Americans

have a special temperament, quite different from North Americans."

"You don't shoot cocaine?"

"Never. Like Freud, I prefer taking my drugs the natural way, orally or by sniffing it."

Leary's smile was cordial but he gazed at the waves of the Pacific, as if our conversation bored him.

"But tell me, Gabe: How can anyone speak intelligently about drugs without having personally experienced them?"

"Would you prevent me from speaking about crime because I'm not a criminal? Do you object if I talk about cancer without suffering from it?" I asked.

"Come on, now. Don't be a sophist, please. There's quite a difference."

"All right then. Since you're recognized, with Dr. Hofmann,[3] as one of the great experts of 'psychedelic' experiments, what is the redeeming value of drugs?"

Tim's well-lined face lit up.

"Let me describe my first experience with psylocibine![4] I was still at Harvard and I was looking for ways to explore the subconscious. After taking a few milligrams of that substance a new vision opened before me. I made an extraordinary journey from which I returned a new man. In four hours I learned more about brain mechanisms and thought processes than during the fifteen previous years."

"When you used a classical experimental methodology?"

"Yes, the kind that produced thousands of studies using psychological and psychiatric tests. But they taught us nothing, Now, with psylocibine, I discovered that the brain is an underused bio-computer, with billions of neurons normally out of reach."

"You say 'normally' but why disrupt the computer to learn about its normal operation? That's rather unusual, as any physiologist will tell you."

Leary shook his head.

"Not at all. I found out, thanks to psylocibine, that our so-called normal consciousness is only a drop in the ocean of knowledge, that consciousness and knowledge can be infinitely expanded and that the brain can be re-programmed."

"Only after it's been de-programmed with a chemical substance that scrambles all its circuits and leaves permanent scars? Your procedure doesn't look too scientific to me, my dear Tim."

"Gabe, you're a slave of objective science and you reject intuitive knowledge generated by these extraordinary substances which affect the mind in deep and mysterious ways! And yet, human beings will control their destiny only if they have a better understanding of the mechanisms of the brain. It's a necessity in the age we live in."

"Agreed, of course, but you can't do it with methods that smack of mental alchemy! You claim there's a magical way to find happiness with substances that poison the brain!"

"You're mistaken, Gabe. You should try these drugs and stop being afraid of them. Become their friend. Join me and my followers and you'll be thrilled to have the key to the wisdom we all aspire to find. I'm only a disciple of Socrates who advised us some two thousand years ago to 'know ourselves.' It is precisely L.S.D. or mescaline, as Aldous Huxley found out, that breaks down the barrier between the conscious and the unconscious. These drugs are perfectly harmless when properly used and allow the user to explore his own psyche. This deepening of the knowledge of the self comes with a mystical vision of the Universe; the world is revealed in its cosmic reality."

The reporters listened to Leary as if they were hearing a present-day prophet. I must admit that there was a spellbinding quality in his words and the serene rhythmic quality of his delivery.

I understood better why he had moved thousands of young people, sensitized by the libertarian revolt of the sixties, to experiment with drugs.

It seemed, however, that Leary's brain had been so deeply affected by L.S.D. that he could no longer make sense. He was incapable of grasping the real dimension of the consumption of substances which impair brain mechanisms and induce circular reasoning. As a result he was unable to distinguish truth from error, right from wrong. He had been hopelessly caught in the trap opened by the brain-altering drugs he had consumed and which had impaired his judgment.

"And now, Tim, what are your plans?"

"Well, until the end of June I'll be on a university lecture tour."

Leary smiled. He appeared supremely happy. After his release from prison he had become a national hero of sorts. He made a very comfortable living by lecturing, mostly with Gordon Liddy, a major figure indicted in the Watergate affair and a strong advocate of conservative causes. The pair, who had met in prison, would debate opposite positions and attract large crowds. Their fee for one appearance reached three thousand dollars plus travel expenses.

"Do you have any plans for the future?" inquired a slim young woman, with half of her face hidden behind saucer-like dark glasses. "Is it true you're going into business?"

"Where did you hear that? Well, yes, I'm starting a computer enterprise in Hollywood: It's called Futique."

"What is 'Futique'?"

"'Futique' is a science turned to the future, the opposite of antique. I've just finished working with computer programmers to create some psychoactive software."

"That sounds like science fiction," I blurted with a laugh.

"Not at all, Gabe! Our software, enclosed in a light fiberglass helmet tightly fitted to the head, emits electro-magnetic wave programs and targets certain brain structures. Some of our programs broaden the field of consciousness, others cause euphoria, others even simulate an L.S.D. psychedelic experience. And it's all caused by signals on various wave lengths. Above all, my dear Gabe, it's perfectly legal!"

He patted my shoulder as the amused crowd looked on.

Leary's declarations were pure inventions. No scientist has ever succeeded in simulating the effects of a drug with electric currents applied to the surface of the skull. It would have been necessary to introduce metal rods inside the brain and stimulate directly the deep areas known as "pleasure and reward" zones. But I had to admit that Leary was not devoid of imagination.

"And now, Tim, how about a story for us?" asked one of the reporters.

Leary looked at me, his blue eyes twinkling with mischief.

"Well, here's a story Gabe should like. One of my prison mates, a notorious member of the Mafia, called his mother one day and told her about the professor who was sharing his cell. 'You mean that Leary who's mixed up with drugs?' said the good woman, 'I'm telling you to stay away from that man. He could get you into trouble.' "

Laughter greeted his words, Leary shook my hand and departed, escorted by an attractive barefooted young woman with long blond hair waving over her swaying form.

"And you, Gabe, what do you think of coke?" asked a reporter.

"I don't agree with Dr. Leary. Cocaine is an extremely dangerous drug."

"More harmful than heroin?"

"Absolutely. It can cause madness, which doesn't happen with heroin."

"Do you believe it is physically addictive?"

"Every study has proven that cocaine modifies the biochemistry of the brain. These are physical changes. Remember the film on the monkey who self-injects cocaine till it dies. The action on the brain induces a behavior of compulsive consumption."

"The film you showed us this morning was very impressive, but humans are not monkeys and they can exercise their free will."

"Yes, except that cocaine breaks will power, robs an individual of the freedom to choose, and enslaves the mind."

"Thank you, doctor."

Ronald Siegel was approaching and the reporters greeted him with the familiarity reserved for the media–anointed experts.

I moved away as I waved Siegel good-bye. He walked over to shake my hand and wish me, with exceeding courtesy and a touch of irony, "A speedy trip back to New York."

"Many thanks," I replied.

I left quickly. I didn't intend to return to Los Angeles and meet again with California's cocaine "experts" who persist in ignoring science and history. Their tolerant attitude towards recreational cocaine use would never stem its epidemic spread.

Nevertheless, I was pleased to have attended the Conference and to have met the Hans Maier of our time, Raoul Jeri. He was the one I wished to see again, in his native land, Peru, a major battleground of the cocaine wars in both ancient and modern times.

My wish was fulfilled less than a year later after I joined an expedition organized by Captain Cousteau to explore the burgeonning cocaine trade in Peru.

IV

THE COCAINE WAR IN PERU: A DEADLOCK

18

Cousteau's Explorers Discover Cocaine in the Amazon Jungle, 1983

In his Paris studio Captain Jacques Yves Cousteau was assembling the first of his films on the Amazon. I had come to visit him in company of another friend, Jacques Constans, a brilliant engineer, polymath and close associate of the captain. Constans had just returned from the Peruvian port of Iquitos near the Brazilian border, high in the Amazon Valley where the Calypso teams[1] were finishing their survey of the planet's largest water basin.

The eagle-featured captain and two of his assistants were assembling clips after projecting them repeatedly on a viewer at various speeds controlled by an operator. Once they had scrutinized the frames, Cousteau and his aides discussed an appropriate spot for splicing them into a section of the film which was, in turn, added to another sequence. Then from hundreds of seemingly unrelated clips Cousteau produced his one hundred and eighty–first film, according to a scenario known to him alone. I was watching a genius at work while he summoned a pageant of living images to reveal the splendid harmony of nature too often devastated by human intrusion.

On the screen, scenes of plant and animal life came alive in a lavish symphony of forms and colors. I viewed a huge flight of red birds wing across a dazzling blue sky above the immense green jungle.

"That'll be the backdrop for the credits of the film," declared Cousteau with satisfaction. "And now, how about lunch?"

At the restaurant, La Mascotte, Jacques Constans, seated next to the captain, explained:

"As I was telling Gabriel, all along the Amazon High

Valley, Indian tribes, pushed and threatened by the cocaine traffickers, give up their traditional manioc crops to grow coca trees."

Cousteau peered at Constans over his half-moon glasses.

"How did that happen?" he asked, "Tribal traditions go back to the dawn of time."

"It started rather recently, about three or four years ago when the traffickers began prospecting the area. At first they met with strong opposition from some tropical forest Indians, such as the Tukanoans. We visited that tribe, where coca used to be considered a sacred substance, and we took some film of the religious rituals where it's consumed in the presence of the tribal shaman. Indians only grew coca for their ceremonies and to communicate with their gods. They planted it sparingly in the middle of their manioc fields following a specific pattern vaguely resembling a human figure."

"So they were bought out?"

"That's it. And today, with the money they get for their coca leaves, the Tukanoans buy aluminum pans, fabrics, tinsel, and even outboard motors for their pirogues. They'll sometimes clear the forest to plant whole groves of coca trees."

"So an actual erosion of the environment is taking place, isn't it?" asked Cousteau, his face sobered.

"You could say that, and worse still," Constans went on. "Coca crops are so profitable that the Indians give up other crops, such as vegetables and manioc, their life staples; they prefer canned goods. Cocaine traffic has created a consumer economy that tends to disrupt their communal tribal life. The elders can't understand why coca, with its divine ritualistic value, is now marketable and lucrative."

"Our Indian has lost his innocence thanks to us, the civilized! And what about cocaine, is it prepared on location?"

"No, not cocaine itself. Only the Indians are learning how to concoct coca paste. They soak the leaves in common chemical products such as kerosene, sulfuric acid, and sodium carbonate, supplied by the traffickers. The mixture is dried in the sun and turns into a yellowish paste with a strong gasoline odor."

"So now the jungle is being chemically polluted," murmured Cousteau. "But what do the Indians do with the paste?"

"Some of it is consumed on location, some sent to the cities where it's smoked. Most of it is airlifted to Colombia where it's processed into cocaine hydrochloride for export to the United States."

I showed the Captain a dossier of American and French press clippings describing the increase in cocaine traffic in North and South America. A series of recent articles from *Le Monde* described the State within a State created by the major drug traffickers in Bolivia where the business community, the state officials, and the farmers have been infiltrated and corrupted, and the country has been destabilized.[2]

Cousteau listened intently and thumbed through the dossier, shaking his head in disbelief.

"In the United States," I told him, "cocaine, a much more harmful drug than heroin, is now used across all social classes. It might be the right time to make a film"

Cousteau was silent and continued to examine the newspaper articles.

Earlier, when the Captain had written the preface for my book, *Keep Off the Grass*,[3] I had suggested that he make a film on drugs. "We'll make one when the time is right," he had answered evasively. He was hesitant to enter an area of controversy, with little inspirational value and quite unrelated to his explorations of oceans and waterways.

"We certainly have the material to make a dynamite documentary," Constans observed.

Finally, Cousteau turned to me:

"Well, talk to Jean-Michel." Jean–Michel is Cousteau's son. "He's in charge of our team of explorers and film producers. They're filming the last stages of the sixth episode on the Amazon. Everything has to be completed by the end of next June. It leaves us barely three months." He shook his head, as if still uncertain.

"We'll have to be very careful. Drug traffickers protect their secret operations with guns."

A few days later, back in New York, I managed to catch Jean-Michel Cousteau between planes at the Cousteau Society offices. Always on the run, he was about to leave for Los Angeles and from there he would fly to join the Calypso team stationed in Lima. With his unkempt beard, his inexhaustible energy, and his quiet efficiency, Jean-Michel is the prototype of the tireless explorer and adventurer. Shaken, as Jacques Constans had been, by the extent of cocaine traffic in the high valleys of the Amazon, he was willing to produce a film on the subject. He had already spoken to Ted Turner, the cable network magnate, who had underwritten the latest Calypso expeditions. Turner was ready to finance a film on cocaine traffic, not included in the original contract.

"I take it that he's also concerned with the problem?"

"He has to face drug use quite often in show business and in the media. I think he's frightened, just like you and all of us, by the ravages of cocaine on his country."

Ted Turner, like many southerners, has a strong loyalty to traditional American values and is critical of the permissive attitudes at some of the large eastern T.V. networks towards recreational illicit drug use.

I mentioned the security problem for the Calypso team, since drug traffickers stop at nothing to protect their clandestine operations.

"Of course" said Jean-Michel. "We'll have to plan and produce the film as discreetly as possible. In any case, we're not in the business of passing judgment. We want to present the facts as they are and make a documentary film. We'll need the support of the government of Peru and the cooperation of their experts, who will be informed of our plans."

I told Jean-Michel I would alert the American Drug Enforcement Agency officials who were working closely with their counterparts in Peru and South America.

"Fine, but your expertise in toxicology is what we particularly need."

I was willing to cooperate, I replied, and even anxious, once in Lima, to call upon the help of Dr. Jeri, the first scientist to study the addiction of young coca paste smokers.

"These unfortunate youth are so addicted and alienated that some Peruvian surgeons have performed lobotomies on them!"

Jean-Michel looked at me with deep concern.

"Did you say 'lobotomy'? Brain surgery?"

"Exactly."

"We'll try to get the operation on film."

A month later I was on the plane to Lima. I had tried to acquaint myself with this land of legends.[4] Nearly twice the size of Texas with a population of twenty million people, Peru holds vast agricultural and mining resources. Located mainly in the tropics, bordered by a fifteen–hundred–mile coastline, split by the high peaks of the Andes, Peru enjoys every type of climate.

The mysterious ruins of the ancient Inca kingdom in Machu-Pichu, high in the mountains, stand as silent remnants of a lost civilization, the first and last indigenous civilization to surface in the Western hemisphere.

In 1823, a vast land stretching from Central America to Chile was liberated from the Spanish colonial yoke by the concerted efforts of San Martin and Simon Bolivar. Reared in France by the Dominicans and trained in Napoleon's entourage, Bolivar died before he could implement institutional reforms which would have cemented the unity of this large territory fragmented by geography and ethnic diversity.

After its liberation from Spain, the new national Peruvian government was dominated by large landowners and remained dependent for its economic development on foreign European nations, mainly Great Britain and France. These countries exploited, for their own profit, the considerable natural resources that Spain had not already exhausted. For more than a century a series of coups and an endless war against Chile tore the country apart, preventing the formation of a national identity crucial to its development. After World War I, the United States stepped in to ensure the economic development of a country dominated by political and military oligarchies locked in a power struggle. Meanwhile, the Indian farmers and miners of the Andes continued to lead the same marginal existence as their forebears and chew their coca leaves, indifferent to the succession of political regimes that had failed to develop the country. Paradoxically, nature and history endowed Peru with all the elements that all great nations are proud to possess: an ancient history, agricultural and mining resources, and a hard-working people.

Nowadays, with the return of a democratic regime following a long military dictatorship, Peru faces a serious economic crisis with a population split between the rich and the *descamisados*. Among the latter, four million Indians, one fifth of the population, most of them coca leaf chewers, live in the five Andean provinces. Moreover, since the end of World War II, a rapid and unplanned industrialization has drawn five million people, one fourth of the population, to Lima. Half of them are jobless and crowded into a city built to house one million.[5]

Karen Brazeau, a seasoned executive of the Cousteau Society and coordinator of the innumerable technical details of "Operation Coca," met me at the airport. As we drove into town I was sickened by the nauseating smell rising from the *favellas,* the mud and scrap iron slums that stretched along the highway to Lima.

Karen warned me:

"Around here, the revolution goes on non-stop, with daily explosions and street riots. It's better not to stray away from our hotel alone — there are a lot of petty thieves around. Besides these minor inconveniences the city is pleasant and the weather remains warm and dry."

The Cousteau team stayed at the Hotel Bolivar, a magnificent structure built around 1900 on the Plaza de la Liberaçion where General San Martin's equestrian statue presides over all the patriotic celebrations.

Once in the hotel lobby, guarded by an unusually high number of muscular doormen, I felt quite secure. In the spacious hall, beveled mirrors reflected tropical plants. Elegantly gowned matrons sipped tea while a musician played Hoffmann's *Barcarolle.* Tourists in sports clothes strolled around, carrying all types of cameras as they prepared to leave for the ruins of the Inca Empire of Cuzco and Machu-Pichu.

Jean-Michel informed me that we would spend a few days in Lima to observe coca paste smokers and study methods used to treat them. From there we would go to see the coca bush plantations of Tingo Maria and Juan Juy in the Upper Amazonian jungle. The next day and for the rest of the expedition we would be joined by Dr. Jeri. He would act as our interpreter and had already scheduled meetings with several Peruvian specialists in the treatment of cocaine addicts.

In the middle of the night a series of loud explosions jolted me out of my sleep. The electricity went off. Although I had been warned that this would happen, I still had to get used to such incidents.

19

When Cocaine Becomes the Religion of a People

Dr. Fernando Cabieses greeted Jean-Michel Cousteau's Calypso crew with extreme courtesy. Heavy-set with a roundish face, graying hair, and a debonair manner, the neurosurgeon, an occasional botanist, could be considered, in Jeri's words, a spokesman for the Peruvian intelligentsia.

Asked for his opinion on the cocaine problem in Peru, he answered without ambiguity:

"First, a fundamental distinction must be made between the cocaine snorted or smoked as a drug, and coca leaves chewed by millions of my compatriots."

"What quantity do they chew?" asked Jean-Michel.

"Andean Indians chew ten grams of leaves at a time in walnut-size balls that they wedge between cheek and gum. With a small stick they add to this ball an alkaline substance made from plant ash and ground chalk. They keep the mixture in their mouths for about forty minutes, a period called a *cocada,* during which they can walk a couple of miles. They chew between three and six of these balls of leaves in a day."

"And why do they add that substance to coca?"

"The alkaline substance, combined with the saliva during the chewing of the leaves, allows a better absorption of cocaine by the mucosa of the mouth. The coca–chewing Indians or *acullicadores* learn how to dose the relative amounts of leaves, chalk, and saliva for the best use of the drug and its desired effects. This isn't just basic chewing, a rumination of sorts, but a learned technique with a high degree of accuracy."

Cabieses spoke English fluently, in quiet, convincing tones. A few precise gestures punctuated his words.

"Are you saying," asked Jean-Michel, "that coca-chewing is socially acceptable but that the use of cocaine isn't?"

"Exactly. Chewing coca is an integral part of the mores of our Andean society. Indians consider coca leaves as a gift from the gods, a symbol of friendship and conviviality."

"How about yourself, do you chew coca leaves?" inquired Jean-Michel.

"Yes, but only when I visit the Indians. I accept the leaves they offer me because it's their way of welcoming me. Sharing coca, consuming it together, is a sign of social integration and human solidarity that binds the participants, just like drinking wine for a toast in your countries."

"But wine doesn't contain alkaloids and is also a food," I remarked.

"The same is true of coca leaves. They contain vitamins, minerals, oils, and other nutritional elements. The Indians chew them in large quantities."

"How large?"

"It depends; between forty and sixty grams a day."

I knew this represented a minute energy intake of about twenty calories. Furthermore, Dr. Cabieses had participated in a study with American scientists who had measured the cocaine concentration in the plasma of coca-chewing Indians.[1] They had found that the quantity of cocaine measured in the blood of these men was comparable to that found in addicts who sniffed pure cocaine in the United States. But this was no time to start an argument with our host.

"Don't forget," added Cabieses, "that coca's medicinal and beneficial effects are well-known to the Indians who use it without abusing it, which can't be said of alcohol with its destructive consequences in western countries, yours for instance. Such damage is a great deal worse than anything caused here by coca."

"So you believe that coca bushes should be grown in Peru?" asked Jean-Michel.

"Absolutely. Indians need coca leaves to live according to their social and cultural traditions. What right do we have to impose our western values and our culture on them?"

"And what would happen if the cultivation of the coca bush was prohibited? In other words, since cocaine is causing so much damage, doesn't it make sense to restrict it at its source?" asked Jean-Michel.

"Unthinkable," declared Cabieses, raising his voice. "Three million Indians would revolt, and this isn't just a guess."

"Have you conducted any studies on the subject?" I asked.

"I haven't, but an American anthropologist, Dr. William Carter, has. Here's his report in a book published by Raoul Jeri in 1981.[2]

Cabieses opened the book.

Listen to Carter's conclusion on page 164:

> A study of two thousand seven hundred and twelve miners working in the Bolivian copper mines of the Altiplano, shows that if coca leaves were not available, forty percent would revolt against the authorities, thirteen percent could no longer work and sixteen percent would become ill. . . . We spent a year with the Andean Indians . . . and we can assert that they are ready to fight the illegal traffic of coca, provided they are allowed to consume their leaves according to their customs. To disregard the Indians' right to use coca would cause a fragmentation of Bolivian society. Furthermore, the white race would once more be guilty of ethnocide.

Cabieses shut the book. The message was clear. Jean-Michel nodded and we exchanged a glance. He knew, as I did, that Jeri's book quoted other medical observations which documented the damaging effects of coca leaf chewing. But we would get to them later.

"One last question," said Jean-Michel. "You're president of the Peruvian Association of Neurosurgeons?"

"I am."

"What do you think of the cyngulotomies performed in your clinic in Lima to treat incurable cocaine addicts?"

Cabieses frowned.

"I can't speak for the Association but I can give you my personal opinion. This operation isn't a new one and has been performed in the past to help incurable addicts. It is premature to claim any results. We lack perspective."

Our host rose and added with a smile, "Before you leave, I would like to show you my hobby: my collection of tropical plants."

We followed him to a large, humid greenhouse where innumerable plants displayed distinctive leaves and blossoms.

"I'm particularly interested in medicinal plants," declared Cabieses. "They contain useful substances, among them the alkaloid extracted from the Erythoxylon Cocalam or Novogranatense, known as cocaine, which is unique in the world. I know of no other remedy that, when properly used, provides greater relief to human suffering. I don't have to tell you, Dr. Nahas, that nothing beats a cocaine solution to induce the best surface anesthesia of the eye or the throat."

"I agree, but without questioning its medical usefulness, it can be replaced."

"And do you know that of the dozens of varieties of Erythoxylon only the two I mentioned contain cocaine?"

"How do you explain, Dr. Cabieses, that among the thousands of Peruvian tropical plants, only the coca bush has reached such a privileged status? It's favored over all the berries, fruit, roots, leaves, or tubers that thrive in your country, including the cocoa bean."

"That's proof enough of the exceptional quality of this substance and the universal power of its appeal."

"Granted, but don't forget its power to enslave humans," I added.

"That's the other side of the coin," said Cabieses. "Roses have thorns."

We received quite a different message from Dr. Manuel Fernandez, head of the department of psychiatry at the University of San Marcos in Lima. He is also in charge of the rehabilitation program for youthful coca paste smokers treated in a specialized Center at the Larco Herera Psychiatric Hospital. This vast building was the first state hospital for the mentally ill built in Lima at the turn of the century. It houses over a thousand patients in two-story structures scattered in a large shaded park.

Fernandez greeted us in front of the pavilion reserved for drug addiction treatment. Tall and portly, with a light complexion, an oval face, and carefully combed black hair, he had the slightly aloof bearing of a Spanish aristocrat.

"This is where we treat about twenty young addicts, former coca paste smokers, *pastaleros*. They're also alcoholics and pot smokers."

"How long do you keep them?" asked Jean-Michel.

"They remain as in-patients for three months and follow a therapy of psychological and physical group rehabilitation we've developed over the last few years. The program consists of sports and educational psychotherapy sessions which I direct with specially trained assistants, doctors, and nurses. Families participate in the treatment."

"You mean parents visit their children?"

"Yes, it's essential because when they leave the hospital, the addicts return home to pursue their rehabilitation. But come and see for yourselves."

A nurse unlocked the heavy entrance door. We crossed a large dining hall that led to a dormitory which opened on a park. A dozen young men were playing soccer as nurses and a few incurable mentally ill old-timers looked on. The youth gathered around Jean-Michel as the camera team started shooting.

The young people seemed in excellent physical condition and responded readily to Jean-Michel's questions. More talkative than the others, a twenty-five year old athlete with some knowledge of English told us that he started smoking marijuana, then moved on to coca paste. He admitted that at one time he smoked eighty cigarettes in a day, one after the other.

"Did you say eighty?" asked Jean-Michel.

"Yes, eighty. But cocaine is garbage, it destroys your brain," he added.

Fernandez informed me, on the side, that this young man was in his third hospital stay and was most recently brought in at the height of a fit of insanity. He was receiving very strong doses of phenothiazines,[3] a medication used in the treatment of schizophrenia.

"I believe his brain is irreversibly damaged."

A seventeen-year-old student admitted having been arrested for holding up a cab to buy coca paste. One of his buddies, he told us, had died in convulsions, "a red foam on his mouth after smoking an awful lot of coca."

A thirty-year-old professor of psychology, married and the father of three, had abandoned his family and his university position. He was only beginning to realize the wreckage he had made of his life. With the help of his wife and of his parents he was determined to recover.

Fernandez escorted us to his office, a large room filled with papers and files stacked high on shelves covering the walls. Seated at his desk, he was ready for an on-camera interview.

"Everybody agrees on the dangers of cocaine, especially

when it is smoked," said Jean-Michel, "but what do you think of the effects of chewing coca leaves?"

Fernandez turned his patrician face towards Jean-Michel.

"There is, of course, no common measure between the two. Coca paste destroys the individual, but coca leaves do not prevent the Indians from working."

"What do we know about the effects of this habit on the health of the Andean Indians?" I asked Fernandez.

Fernandez smiled lightly.

"You're touching a very controversial subject. I'll give you my opinion, shared by my colleagues Guterriez Noriega and Zapata Ortiz, two specialists in that area. The three million Indians from the Altiplano live in dire poverty.[4] They are, for the most part, illiterate and suffer from malnutrition. They show a high incidence of acute parasitical, infectious, and chronic diseases, such as heart, kidney, and circulatory ailments. Frequent cases of dwarfism, cretinism, and congenital malformations have been reported. Jeri could certainly complete the picture for you."

"Neurological disorders of all kinds have been observed," supplied Jeri. "But it is difficult to attribute them to coca. We lack parallel studies of populations living under similar conditions in non-coca chewing cultures."

I mentioned the case of the Tibetans who, like the Andeans, live at high altitudes. They do not use drugs and are solid mountain climbers who have developed a mystical culture with a world-wide following.

"That could make a fine research project in comparative anthropology," I suggested.

"Probably, but in the meanwhile," continued Fernandez, "our Indians vegetate with their coca and there's been no improvement in their living conditions in the five hundred years since the Spanish conquest!"

This was recognized by the 9th Session of the International Commission on Narcotics in April of 1954. Representatives of Peru, Bolivia, Colombia, and Argentina recognized that coca chewing constitutes a harmful form of drug addiction.

"It has been established," confirmed Jeri, "that the *coqueros* chew thirty to sixty grams of coca leaves a day, which represents a dose of three to six hundred milligrams of cocaine.

Furthermore, studies of coca chewers by the American scientist Byck and by our own Dr. Cabieses reported cocaine blood concentrations of several hundred nanograms per milliliter.[5] Such concentrations disrupt brain functions and are similar to those measured in American cocaine sniffers who use the drug for the sole purpose of getting high. The normal state of a coca chewer is a permanent high, but he will not present the severe symptoms of the pastalero who absorbs in half an hour the daily dose of a *coquero.*"

"But isn't it true that Peruvians chewed coca long before the Spanish arrived?" asked Jean-Michel.

"Indeed. I'd like to point out that due to the climate, coca was grown exclusively on the eastern slopes of the Andes and in a few coastal towns. Those areas were quite inaccessible and distant from those where the Incas, the potential consumers, used to live. They were also at some distance from the present settlement of the Altiplano Indians."

"And you conclude what from this?" asked Jean-Michel.

"Three things. First, coca use in Peru was probably quite limited before Pizarro's arrival. Secondly, its use spread during the periods of religious and political unification which fostered the economic and commercial development of the country. Finally, the trivialization of coca use among the natives occurred after the Spanish conquest."

"And in spite of the opposition of the Church and the Viceroy Francisco de Toledo," added Jeri.

"If this habit is as debilitating as you claim, do you think the use of coca could be prohibited in Peru?" asked Jean-Michel.

"In the immediate future, there isn't a chance. The use of coca is too deeply rooted in Andean culture where it constitutes a genuine ritual. Indians chew it at work, during meals, at all traditional ceremonies, marriages, baptisms, funerals. . . . "

"Then what could make them give it up?"

"An acceptable alternative, a new social order. If not, the Indians would experience a 'social withdrawal syndrome,' to use the language of pharmacology."

"You mean they would revolt?"

"Indeed. To prohibit the growing of the coca bush would lead to an economic breakup of the country. Farmers would have to be compensated and receive help in establishing substitute crops that would be far less lucrative for them than cocaine."

Dr. Fernandez' compassionate expression hardened as he raised his voice:

"Deep economic and social changes would be necessary, and they're hard to implement presently in our country whose conservative economic policies are supported by the United States."

"So you don't see any possibility of decreasing the production of coca?"

"Unfortunately not," answered Fernandez. "Today we can only cope with urgent situations and save a few of the young people who are hooked on cocaine."

"They seem to be on the way to recovery," remarked Jean-Michel.

"Yes, as long as they stay in this sheltered environment, they progress remarkably and relate once more to family members who visit them. When they leave us, they're still very vulnerable and they're liable to fall into their old habits."

"What's the relapse rate?"

"In the last six years, since the Center was started, eighty percent of our patients relapse within a year of their release."

"And how long do they stay with you?"

"Three months. It's too short, but government funds are limited, and a bed shortage keeps us from lengthening a patient's stay. We have waiting lists! Anyway, after three months, all these young people are anxious to get out and resume their activities. We need workshops, vocational training centers where we can organize athletic programs and group psychotherapy. As soon as the *pastaleros* leave the hospital they're back in an environment where drugs are everywhere."

"Repeated relapses have led some of your colleagues to perform surgical operations on the brain. What's your position on this?" asked Jean-Michel.

Fernandez' mood turned grave.

"That method reminds me of those I saw in Anthony Burgess' film *Clockwork Orange* to reprogram deviant individuals. Similarly, we've heard that brainwashing is practiced in mental wards in the USSR. But we mustn't forget that psychosurgery has been prohibited in that country because of the danger of its use when applied to political opponents."

I added that Western Europe no longer practices that kind of surgery.

"In any case," continued Jeri, who seemed anxious to change the subject, "Dr. Fernandez is doing a fine job, but his Center is overcrowded."

"Is it the only center in Lima?"

"No, other government centers provide an additional hundred beds, and there are about a hundred more beds in private clinics."

"And how many *pastaleros* need treatment?"

"Two years ago" responded Jeri, "I conducted a survey for the Health Ministry and estimated that there were a hundred thousand in Lima."

As we left the hospital, our taxi drove by a white van with the name SANDOZ painted in large black letters. The Peruvian branch of this international drug company was delivering a shipment of phenothiazines, powerful tranquilizers in the treatment of schizophrenia.

Jeri leaned toward me.

"Fernandez musn't be too happy to see this truck on his territory."

"Why?'

"Because he doesn't believe that multinational companies should get rich at the expense of developing countries."

"But Sandoz allows schizophrenic patients to return home and make room for *pastaleros* who need to be treated."

"That's true, but you surely noticed Fernandez has been influenced by revolutionary ideas."[6]

"Regardless," I reflected, "in the Peruvian Andes, religion is no longer 'the opium of the people' as Karl Marx once claimed. Rather, opium, or more precisely, cocaine has become the religion of the people."

"But the coca war is also a religious war," retorted Jeri, "right here and also in your own country!"

20

Treating the *Pastaleros* With Astronaut's Vitamins

Notified by Raoul Jeri of the visit of the Cousteau team, Dr. Nizama Valladolid was most anxious to meet us and have a chance to record on film his new treatment for coca paste addicts. The affable young psychiatrist, short, dark, round-faced, ushered us into his office on the second floor of an elegant building in the district of Miraflores, a residential area with wide tree-lined avenues.

Jean-Paul Cornu, the photographer, set up his spotlights, and Nizama began his presentation, speaking briskly, with self-assurance, as if he were lecturing to his students.

He first displayed some samples of the coca paste found on his patients: "As you can see, it is a brownish powder, wrapped in square pieces of newspaper of various sizes. The smallest dose is called a 'gunshot' by the dealers. Then comes the 'cannon ball,' and finally the largest one is the 'Exocet,' named after the French missile which sank that English battleship during the Falklands war."

"Basic coca paste," he went on, "is smoked in an ordinary cigarette. Shreds of tobacco are removed from the tip and replaced with paste. Those who smoke this mixture soon become slaves of their habit and center their whole lives around the drug."

"Confronted with the failure of all the therapies now in use, I conceived and tested a new method. It combines modern anti-cocaine chemotherapy with a restructuring of the addict's personality. Associated with group psychotherapy and support from the family, this treatment restores the cocaine addict to a normal behavior acceptable to his kin and to society."

"What type of chemotherapy do you use?" I asked.

"Thorazine and also Haldol."[1]

These powerful substances are used in the treatment of schizophrenia, the most severe form of mental illness.

"But your patients aren't schizophrenics," I commented.

"They may not be, but when they're on a coca paste binge, they present every symptom of schizophrenia: delirium, hallucinations, irresponsible compulsive behavior."

"And what dose do you prescribe?"

"Between two and three hundred milligrams a day of thorazine and three to five milligrams of Haldol."

"In combination?"

"Yes, it's much more effective."

Such doses seemed massive to me. They are prescribed by psychiatrists, for short periods, to treat the most severe cases of schizophrenia.

"And how do you manage to make them take such strong doses on a regular basis?"

"We rely on the parents' help. They mix the medication in the food and increase or decrease the doses according to their children's behavior."

Jean-Michel shook his head, a gesture noticed by Nizama, who explained:

"In Peru, though family ties are very strong, they can be destroyed by cocaine. We have seen the rise of a pathetic new type of delinquency: family delinquency: the cocaine addict becomes a thief within his own family. He steals from his parents, brothers, sisters, because he knows they won't turn him in to the police. First he sells his own personal belongings and then goes on to sell his family's. Everything goes: Jewels, silverware, art objects, furniture, and even linen. Addicts have been known to assault their parents, physically abuse their mothers and their sisters. When we treat them, we ask for the family's help. But I'd like you to meet some of my patients."

Five young men walked slowly into the room and sat down facing the camera. The similarity of their behavior struck me: same automatic and jerky gestures, same pale frozen faces at times twitched by tics. One of them constantly inflated and deflated his cheeks, another stuck his tongue out intermittently, while another would open and then close his mouth off and on. Their hands and their fingers trembled slightly but continuously, as they do in many old people.

These symptoms could be attributed to the large doses of phenothiazines or tranquilizing medications administered, which are known to produce biochemical changes in certain brain areas that coordinate all of the signals required for muscle relaxation. Such manifestations are called tardive dyskinesias: Tardive because they are usually observed only after prolonged treatment of schizophrenic patients, and their occurrence is considered a serious complication which mandates either interruption of therapy or marked decrease in dosage.

We were in the presence of former cocaine addicts, doped with enormous doses of tranquilizers which turned them into docile, infantile persons also affected as a result of this treatment by the trembling of old age.

Nizama addressed one of his patients:

"Pedro, tell us your story."

"I'm eighteen. Two years ago, one day after school, I tried drugs with some friends."

"You mean you started smoking coca paste?" asked Nizama.

"Yes, that's it, and I kept on doing it."

He spoke in a listless, droning voice.

"I couldn't stop. I didn't have enough money, so I started stealing from my parents, my grandparents, my brothers. Then I ran away from home and tried to rob a cabdriver with a toy pistol. I was arrested and they sent me back home because I was a minor. But all I wanted to do was smoke coca paste. So my parents brought me here, to Dr. Nizama."

"And now, what?" asked the doctor.

"Oh, since I'm being treated by Dr. Nizama, I don't want to smoke coca paste any more and I'm living at home with my family."

"Thanks, Pedro," said Nizama. "I could go on questioning these youngsters, but their stories are all very much like Pedro's. They usually come from educated, well-to-do families, so they follow my treatment with the support of their relatives. They lead a very structured life in their homes and follow a program I have conceived. They're assigned readings from great authors and philosophers such as Cervantes, St. John of the Cross, and Shakespeare. Every day they write essays on their reading and keep a log of their own thoughts and ideas.

Nizama showed us a stack of notebooks. As I glanced at them, I noticed the fine, shaky handwriting, a result of the tremor in their fingers caused by the huge amounts of medication they were absorbing.

"And now," said Nizama, "let's meet their parents."

The parents replaced their children, facing the camera lights. Dressed simply, ill at ease, these people belonged to the middle class. A gray-haired man in his fifties, with whom Jean-Michel could converse in English, spoke out.

"We're a group of parents who meet every Monday. We come from about fifty families. The problem we're facing is dreadful, really dreadful."

His voice broke down.

"May I ask you a personal question?" inquired Jean-Michel.

"Of course."

"Tell me, when you found out that your son was a drug addict, what did you do? Do you think you did the right thing?"

"Well, it was four years ago. I discussed the situation with doctors and priests. 'Your son,' they pointed out, 'is twenty-four. He's a man, and you're no longer responsible for his actions.' So I ordered my son out of the house."

"You actually threw him out?"

"Yes, to force him to work. But it was a disastrous decision."

"You think it was the wrong move?"

"Yes, it was. The remedy I chose only aggravated the disease. My son became a human ruin. He was lost."

The man's voice broke down again.

"I understand," said Jean-Michel softly. "And now your son is taking medication without knowing it."

The father shrugged:

"It's true, he knows nothing, absolutely nothing. We tell him he's taking vitamins, the kind they use in Houston for astronauts."

"Vitamins for astronauts?"

"Right, vitamins for astronauts. Our child was lost, remember. Dr. Nizama gave him back to us."

21

Cocaine Addiction and Psychosurgery

Our cab pulled up in front of number 460 Bolognesi Avenue, the Heidelberg Clinic, a large brick residence in the fashionable neighborhood of Miraflores.

The director of the clinic, Dr. Theobaldo Llosa, welcomed us at the entrance. Tall, slightly stooped, with his thin face, high forehead, light complexion and somewhat somber mein; he appeared to be of recent Spanish descent.

"Let me show you our facilities while the camera crew sets up its equipment in the garden. After that, I will be glad to answer your questions."

The Heidelberg Clinic, a large private home formerly owned by one of Lima's first families, had been remodeled into a psychiatric establishment.

"We have twenty-three beds for in-patients. We perform electroshock treatments and sleep therapy. We also treat cocaine addicts who are potential candidates for a cyngulotomy. I'd like you to meet a patient who underwent the operation a year ago."

He led us to a room where a dark-haired young woman was lying on a bed with an intravenous infusion in her forearm.

"Benita," he asked, "Could I show the scar of your operation to my colleagues?"

She acquiesced and leaned forward. Llosa gently parted the woman's hair to reveal a white scar that ran along the hairline.

"And why is she hospitalized?"

"She came for her Vitamin B perfusion."

He pointed to the flask, filled with a bright yellow solution, hanging from a stand at the foot of the bed.

"You see," he explained, "she's an alcoholic with incipient neurological problems.[1] She's an out-patient and she'll leave the clinic after her treatment. You may talk to her."

The young woman spoke in Spanish very freely with Raoul Jeri, who translated her story for us as it unfolded.

She had started smoking coca paste four years before with some friends, to find out what it was like and for the fun of it. Before coca she had tried marijuana and was drinking a lot because she liked what it did for her. "You feel relaxed and you forget your worries."

Once she started on coca paste, she couldn't stop. She ran away from home and lived in a commune with other *pastaleros* for several months before her family located her. She went through several detoxification treatments, including "sleep therapy." She was put to sleep for the best part of two weeks with hypnotics. Nothing worked, and she kept going back to coca paste. She even turned to religion and stayed in a convent for a while, but to no avail. In the end, her parents took her to the Heidelberg Clinic where she agreed to the operation. That was a year ago and she hadn't touched coca paste since. She didn't even miss it any more, and her life was back to normal.

"And what's your occupation?" asked Jean-Michel.

"I'm a student at the university."

"And what are you studying?"

"Psychology and social sciences."

From her conversation, this young woman seemed in full control of her intellectual faculties and suffered no neurological after-effects.

"How old is she?" I asked.

"Twenty-two—and she comes from a fine family," answered Llosa as he led us to other parts of the clinic, occupied by schizophrenic and manic depressive patients attended by nurses in immaculate white uniforms.

We walked again past the room of the young girl we had spoken to earlier and noticed her bed was empty.

"She just left on her motorcycle," Llosa told us.

Back in the garden, Llosa sat under the shade of a spreading tree dotted with scarlet blossoms and answered Jean-Michel's questions in front of the camera.

"First, I must tell you that we don't operate on all the patients who are brought to us, far from it," stated Llosa. "They undergo a rigorous screening. We only select hopeless cases of cocaine addiction who are referred to us by their desperate families. These addicts are also declared untreatable by conventional methods after being examined by a team of psychiatrists, neurologists, and psychologists."

"And what's your criteria when you classify them as 'untreatable?' "

"There are four: first the *pastaleros* must have been smoking coca continuously for two years at least. Secondly, they've attempted several times to quit and never succeeded."

"They relapsed after each treatment?"

"Exactly. Thirdly, they've all been, repeatedly and unsuccessfully, four times on the average, through special treatments, either with Professor Fernandez at the Larco Herrera Hospital or with Dr. Nizama and his psychopharmacological method. Finally, the progressive mental and physical deterioration recognized by their families has been confirmed through medical examinations."

"You consider these criteria sufficient to perform that kind of surgery?"

"Yes," answered Llosa without hesitation. "We estimate they allow us to reach what doctors call a 'prognosis fatalis,' or a diagnosis of imminent death. Let me repeat, this prognosis is based on the recognition that all known treatments have failed and that, abandoned to himself, the *pastalero* will continue to deteriorate, to break his parents' hearts, to become a chronic delinquent, and to suffer acute psychotic crises that will end in murder or suicide. In many cases mothers will tell us: 'I'd rather see my child dead than in this state.' "

"Don't you think these *pastaleros* might have, from the beginning, a marked tendency towards compulsive behavior?"

"Some years ago many cocaine users presented a depressive or a psychotic disposition and the young *pastaleros* often came from unstable or broken homes. Nowadays, it's quite different! *Pastaleros* come from all social groups, rich or poor, educated or illiterate, from happy or unhappy families."

"That's what Dr. Nahas has been telling us," declared Jean-Michel, glancing at me. "Cocaine attracts all types and doesn't distinguish between different brains."

"It's a fact," continued Llosa. "Furthermore, we know that cocaine has the same hold on the adolescent and the adult. It used to be that spouses brought their wives or husbands to our clinic; now we see children bring their own parents."

"Could you tell us more about this so-called 'psychosurgical' operation, as you call it?" asked Jean-Michel.

"The principle isn't new: it's an attempt to decrease the impulses that prevail in the emotional limbic brain, while increasing the power of the new brain in control of rational behavior. Here, let me explain how it works. Cocaine chemically stimulates a fundamental brain mechanism that triggers sensations of reward and pleasure each time hunger, thirst, or love-making, to take a few examples, have been gratified. The purpose of psychosurgery is to partly sever the transmission lines that connect the pleasure centers located in the old brain to the cortex area of the new brain which controls rational and voluntary actions."

"In other words," said Jean-Michel, "the purpose is to decrease the dominance of instincts and impulses over behavior. It's a kind of manipulation of the transmission lines of the brain."

"If you wish. In any case, the hypothesis and the resulting operation are not new. It was performed a hundred years ago by the Swiss surgeon Buckhardt,[2] and later in 1936 by Professor Moniz,[3] who was awarded a Nobel Price jointly with the Swiss neurophysiologist Hess."

"Could you describe the operation for us?"

"A portion of the nerve fibers of the white matter of the frontal brain are severed. These fibers form a cluster, the cyngulus, which surrounds the mid-section of the brain, on each side of the brain hemispheres."

"And how is it actually done?"

"There are several procedures. Originally the fibers were sectioned somewhat blindly by introducing in the brain metal probes that entered the skull either near the temples by 'prefrontal leucotomy,'[4] or near the upper level of the orbits of the eye by 'preorbital leucotomy.' In 1953, the French neurosurgeon Le Beau[5] developed a more precise procedure: the anterior bilateral cyngulotomy; after trepanation the cyngulum is exposed in full view and can be sectioned with precision. We use that method."

"Has this type of surgery been performed by others before you?"

"Yes, it used to be the only way incurable obsessional psychoses could be stabilized or even cured before drugs like phenothiazines became available. This operation did not modify the emotional life of the patient, who could often resume a normal existence. Thousands of operations were performed in India,[6] England,[7] France,[8] and the United States[9] until the mid 1970's."

"Only on the mentally ill?"

"No, this operation was also performed on amputees who suffered the same kind on uncontrollable pain as Von Fleishl, Freud's friend who was first addicted to morphine and then to cocaine.[10] After a cyngulotomy, some patients were able to give up morphine without suffering from withdrawal symptoms. These observations prompted us to try the same operation on cocaine addicts."

"Your team performed it first?"

"Yes, on cocaine addicts. Other groups did it before us, on morphine addicts."[11]

"And what are the possible side-effects of these operations?"

"Neurological complications are negligible. During the immediate post–operative period, convulsions may occur, and they are controlled with short-term anti–convulsive medications."

"What about emotional or psychological side-effects?"

"As you may have observed in speaking to the young woman we saw, there are no in-depth personality changes; intellectual capacities remain intact, as do tactile, visual, auditory, and sensory perceptions. Emotionally, the patients are more subdued, but I find their level of sensitivity quite normal. After their operation they lead normal emotional and sexual lives."

"Then why are you so harshly criticized by your colleagues in psychiatry and in the medical world in general?"

"It's a sign of our times. Many psychiatrists are ill-informed and influenced by a speculative psychoanalytical ideology, completely removed from neurophysiology and psychopharmacology. To them, the *word* reigns supreme. They believe that endless discourses can modify behavior. And yet everyone knows that 'logotherapy' does not cure addiction."

"Some psychiatrists have accused you of applying methods reminiscent of those used by the Nazis."

Llosa was hurt by the remark and shook his head sadly.

"I know," he sighed, " they're just ignorant. What else can they offer the unfortunate *pastaleros* and their families besides words? Without the operation, most of these creatures are doomed to die within a short time."

Dr. Llosa handed me a report he planned to present before the Seventh International Meeting of Psychiatrists in Vienna the following summer.[12] It contained a summary of the twenty-eight case histories of cocaine addicts which had been "cyngulotomized" in Lima over the past two years. Half of them had reinserted themselves into society and were no longer using coca although it was widely available. These results were conclusive enough to encourage Drs. Llosa and Hinojosa to continue operating on selected cases of cocaine addiction in the absence of any other alternative.

And Llosa concluded:

"We are confronted with compulsive behavior resulting from the action of cocaine on the brain. This behavior will eventually kill the victim living in a society where the drug is freely available. We are physicians first, and we are trying to treat an incurable disease by methods based on neuro-pathology. Until now our results have been positive in fifty percent of the cases."

I learned that the operation costs about two thousand dollars, a substantial sum which only wealthy Peruvians can afford.

I was reminded of the trepanations frequently performed by the Shamans — Peruvian medicine men — one thousand years ago. At the Museum of Anthropology of Lima I had observed on several mummies the gaping openings in the skulls of precolombian skeletons.

I was struck by the extent of bone damage of the operated skulls: round or square jagged perforations, from one to three inches wide, surrounded by an area where the bone was made bare to prepare for the operation. As the French anatomist Paul Broca[13] had already noted in 1867, the surgery was done in two stages. The surgeon first removed a piece of scalp at least twice as large as the planned aperture. Then he cut into the bone and excised a round or square section. He used a special gold or brass instrument, a "Tumi," which is one of the national emblems of Peru. It consists of a sharp half-moon blade attached to a rounded handle about four inches long. In some cases, the edge of the bone was porous, suggesting a post-operation infection; sometimes a "cal" scar tissue rimmed the opening, indicating the patient survived for several weeks or months. After the trepanation, the shaman did not section the meninges, membranes that surround the brain, thus keeping it protected. One wonders what kind of anesthesia was available. Some anthropologists have suggested the local application of cocaine paste, combined with the administration of fermented drinks. To avoid an infection the shaman probably applied to the wound the famous "Peruvian Balm," a mixture of salt, menthol, tanin, and saponines, all astringent and antiseptic products.

In some mass graves one skull out of six had been perforated, an indication that trepanations were common in ancient Peru, while seldom performed nowadays in developed countries. No ancient civilization has left as many traces of a practice already in existence during the Stone Age for ritualistic reasons. For example, in ancient Egypt surgeons seldom resorted to trepanation and even guarded against it in their medical writing.[14]

Most of the trepanated skulls which have been examined in Peru do not show signs of fractures or lesions which could justify surgical intervention: a ritual act appears the more likely explanation.[15] It appears possible that evil spirits were being let out of the head of epileptics or of demented individuals, some of whom, who knows? may have suffered from a cocaine psychosis. It is also plausible that trepanations, at first a strictly ritual practice performed by well-trained shamans, later found therapeutic applications, for instance in cases of crushed skulls.

One may wonder if the present-day Peruvian surgeons who perform cyngulotomies to free the cocaine addict from an unrelenting dependency are not repeating a ritual enacted by their ancestors a thousand years ago.

According to the latest report of Dr. Theobaldo Llosa[16] this is certainly not the case. Six years after our first encounter, in 1989 I met him again at the annual PRIDE meeting. Llosa informed me that a follow-up study of 30 patients operated on in Lima between 1981 and 1983 had shown that 18 of them (60% of the group) were drug-free 5 to 7 years after the operation. The recovered addicts were leading useful lives and held steady jobs; some had families. None of them presented neurologic or psychiatric after-effects from their brain surgery. Dr Llosa claimed that these results vindicated the usefulness of psychosurgery in the treatment of irreversibly-addicted cocaine users, and so he and his group are again performing cyngulotomies on what they call the "irrecoverables." He declared:

> In the course of our seven-year follow-up period we have not become aware of a more effective therapeutic procedure than psychosurgery. . . . I believe that one day it will be a therapeutic method of choice in the United States.

I attempted to temper the enthusiasm of Dr. Llosa by informing him that the medical consensus in the United States and Europe was still opposed to this type of operation even for "irrecoverable addicts." Furthermore, the drug-free therapeutic communities that claim similar success after a long residential stay would also strongly object. For me, the resumption of such drastic procedures was indicative of cocaine's widespread use and availability in Peru and of the fact that coca paste smoking had become trivialized in Lima. These foreboding facts indicate that the Peruvian authorities are unable to control the plague and urgently require outside help.

22

Tingo Maria: The White City

With my camera pressed against the window of an AIR PERU plane I was taking pictures of the Altiplano,[1] an arid plateau surrounded by deep valleys that stretches between the two chains of the Andes separating Lima from Tingo Maria. Nestled at the foot of the western slopes of the mountains, in the heart of coca-growing country, the small town of Tingo Maria is known as "the white city" because it has become the most important cocaine traffic center in Peru. We traveled under the watchful eyes of the Peruvian police, escorted throughout our trip by a young officer, Captain Ramon Villades. He had joined us the day before and warned us of danger ahead. The liaison officer from the American Drug Enforcement Agency had advised Jean-Michel against venturing into an area where the drug lords laid down the law. The plane began its descent over the rounded crests of mountains covered with a luxuriant vegetation. Captain Ramon pointed through the window at pale green patches dotting the dark green of the jungle.

"Coca plantations." He smiled.

We spotted the small Tingo Maria airport at the foot of a large wooded hill called "The Sleeping Woman" because its crestline forms a contour like that of a reclining woman.

Four police agents were waiting for us with two vans stationed in front of a somewhat primitive air terminal. Colonel Diomedes Vargas, a large muscular man built like a boxing champion, hurried us along to his car.

"Let's not hang around here where everyone can see us. My men will take care of your luggage."

Our driver raced down the road mindless of potholes, jostling and shaking us until we reached the Peruvian Police

Force headquarters (PPF), a one-story prefabricated building located on the outskirts of town. On one of the walls a black scrawl, "Death to the PPF," had been partly whitewashed. The police force, trained by American agents, was primarily in charge of the repression of cocaine traffic.

"They're equipped with light firearms and four-wheel traction vehicles," Jeri told us, "some armoured, but inadequate against the traffickers' armament, which we are told even includes portable missiles."

Colonel Vargas informed us that there had been some arrests that morning, and he offered to re-enact them for us. He seemed exceedingly anxious to demonstrate the efficiency of his men in front of the cameras. The equipment was promptly in place, and Jean-Paul Cornu began shooting with his usual skill. Two young women with babies in their arms walked down a shaded road full of puddles. Suddenly two husky men in civilian garb approached them and whisked them off to the police station. They found two bags of coca paste hidden in their clothes.

The youngest one, an unwed mother of seventeen with attractive regular features and long dark hair, breastfed her four month old baby. She told us that a stranger had given her seventy-five dollars to take the coca paste to Lima and bring it to someone she didn't know. She took the bus with her friend who was also carrying a bag. They would have spent twenty-five hours on the road!

"Does this woman know that she could get ten to fifteen years in jail for coca traffic?" asked Jean-Michel.

When the question was translated the woman covered her eyes and started sobbing.

"No, I didn't know," she whispered.

As for her friend, she was aware of the risks but claimed she had no other choice. The five–month child she was carrying was her last born. She had four more back home and her husband had left her for another woman. She desperately needed money to feed her brood.

The latest arrivals joined the other women prisoners in a large communal cell, closed on one side by tall iron bars and opening on an inner court. The young woman gently placed her baby on the ground, kneeled down, and changed him. Through the bars I could see the baby smile.

On the opposite side of the courtyard, some thirty feet away, the men's prison was packed. A few prisoners were lying on the ground; others stood and leaned against the wall or the iron bars of the cell. The men were barely able to move about in the cramped quarters, and the pungent smell emanating from such a concentration of bodies rose in the heavy moist heat of the stifling compound.

Colonel Vargas ushered us into his office, a bare room with a table and two chairs.

On a large map pinned to the wall he pointed out the areas where the coca bushes grow: in the valleys along the River Huallaga, from Tingo Maria to Juan Juy, two hundred miles north.

"In this area," he told us, tracing a circle on the map with his finger, "the climate and the volcanic soil combine to yield six crops a year."

"Did you say six?"

"Yes, sir, I did, which is a huge yield, more than half a ton per acre. Most of the coca produced in Peru, for legal or illegal purposes, comes from this area."

"But at that rate, it won't be long before the soil is depleted, especially without fertilizers."

Vargas nodded.

"That's the great pity of our land. First deforestation to plant coca trees, then depletion of the soil that robs future generations."

"And what is your responsibility?"

"Keep track of the growers."

"How large is the cultivated area?"

Vargas chased an insect away from his face.

"The cultivated area must cover between one hundred and twenty-five and one hundred and fifty thousand acres. But the coca plantations aren't all adjacent. They're scattered among other plantations in the jungle, on an acreage that could be a hundred times larger."

"And how do you keep track of such a wide area?"

"We have a hundred men stationed between Tingo Maria and Juan Juy on roads that follow the river. In addition, we have vans like the one you took, and radio communications."

"What more do you need?" asked Jean-Michel.

"We need helicopters, light planes, outboard motorboats,

radar. But the Americans who finance us assume, rightly so, that we wouldn't be able to service this type of equipment properly. In our climate engines deteriorate rapidly."

"What about the traffickers?"

"They've got fast planes and much more powerful arms than ours. They have bazookas while we have rifles and machine guns."

"Is the total figure of the coca crop in Peru known?"

"It's very difficult to estimate with any precision since most of the crops end up in illegal trading. But by regrouping information from various sources—we manage to get an idea of the extent of the harvests."

"And how large are they?" I asked.

"In Peru, the largest producer of coca in South America, the cultivated area is approximately a hundred and seventy-five thousand acres. In Bolivia it's about a hundred and forty thousand acres. To these figures you add the illegal plantations in Colombia, Brazil, and Ecuador, which were started in the last few years. There are also some in Venezuela and Argentina, but fewer. All in all, you have some three hundred and seventy-five thousand acres yielding a ton of leaves per two and a half acres, which in turn produce about six hundred tons of coca paste per year or over two hundred tons of cocaine. The plantations are scattered in remote areas, difficult to reach and spread over one fifth of the continent of South America."

"Practically impossible to patrol!"

Vargas nodded.

"All our armed forces couldn't do the job! Especially since Bolivia and Peru have legalized some plantations to satisfy the needs of the Indian population."

Colonel Vargas then led us to a two-story whitish stucco building that housed E.N.A.C.O.,[2] the national monopoly in charge of managing the legal coca crops that supply the leaves chewed by the Indians and those used to make cocaine for medical purposes.

The Director, a short, balding, and slightly overweight man, greeted us with ingratiating courtesy, withheld, however, from Colonel Vargas.

"All our crops are carefully regulated," he assured us. Every tree is numbered and registered. Each farmer receives a special permit indicating the number of plants he's authorized to grow."

"And how much do you harvest annually?"

"We harvest thirty thousand tons of leaves for the Indians of the Altiplano, and we export twenty thousand tons to the United States, where a cocaine-free extract is made to flavor your famous Coca Cola. The quantities earmarked for medical use are relatively small: approximately one thousand tons of leaves."

"And how much cocaine does a ton or a ton and a half of leaves produce?" asked Jean-Michel.

"In round figures, to estimate the quantity of coca paste obtained from leaves, you divide their weight by two hundred and fifty. To get the quantity of cocaine you divide by six hundred and twenty-five."

"It's rather complicated," remarked Jean-Michel.

"Not at all," retorted the director. "A simple division."

He wrote the figures on a pad: "A ton of coca leaves, or a thousand kilos, divided by two hundred and fifty, you get four kilos of coca paste. The same quantity, divided by six hundred and twenty-five, you get one point six kilos (three and a half pounds) of cocaine powder."

"The yield of the operation is rather high," concluded Jean-Michel.

"Certainly, but at E.N.A.C.O. we're particularly interested in research on the beneficial effects of cocaine. Taken in moderate doses, it's one of the best medications known to the world."

"Do you really think so?" I asked.

"It's not my opinion. I'm quoting Professor Weil of Harvard University."

The director handed me a copy of an article signed by Andrew Weil, dated 1981, entitled "The Therapeutic Value of Cocaine in Contemporary Medicine," which appeared in the Journal of Ethnopharmacology,[3] published in the United States.

A medical student at Harvard during the sixties, Andrew Weil became an advocate of the recreational use of natural coca extracts, and his article, reprinted by E.N.A.C.O., concluded:

Coca is very useful in the treatment of gastro-intestinal infections, walking difficulties and diseases of the larynx. It can be prescribed to lose weight, increase physical stamina and as an anti-depressant. Cocaine also provides a support treatment for addicts hooked on more powerful drugs. Coca is a unique regulator of sugar metabolism and can be very useful to treat diabetes and hypoglycemia. In small doses cocaine appears to stabilize all physiological functions. The untreated leaves are not toxic and not habit-forming.

I handed the piece back to the director, who refused it. "Oh no, you may keep it," he said. "You see, we're hoping that research by scientists like you will find new therapeutic uses for coca. We could then legally develop its cultivation. It would be the best way to fight illicit traffic." I did not answer, while Vargas muttered and Jean-Michel asked Jeri to thank the director for all of us.

Night was falling as we left the sultry premises of E.N.A.C.O.

"I can't stand this bureaucrat," said Vargas, "all he thinks about is how to justify greater areas of coca cultivation. As if there was not enough!"

Vargas then warned us it would be dangerous to spend the night at the hotel, known as a den of well–armed, trig-ger–happy traffickers, foes of any visiting film-makers. "Every day on the streets of Tingo, we find bodies nobody claims."

The Colonel suggested we spend the night at the Francis-can Mission on the edge of town. He assured us we would be perfectly safe there, especially since Captain Ramon would be staying with us. The Canadian Franciscans had built the mis-sion like a small colonial fort, at the center of a quadrangle of walls three feet thick and sixteen feet high. The good Fathers gave us a friendly greeting and assigned each one of us to a monastic cell. Night fell suddenly around six, as it does in the tropics, bringing cool air to relieve us from the sultriness of the day.

"Now you can go to town," said the Father Abbot. "I advise you to stay within the limits of the shopping district. About five hundred yards from there, you'll find a restaurant. Be sure you stay away from a neighborhood called Pequeno Chicago [Little Chicago]." He added grimly, "It's very, very bad."

He handed over the keys of the mission's large gateway to Jean-Michel. Our little troop left the shelter of the Franciscan fortress to venture into town along rutted streets. The shabby stores displayed the latest models in radios, cameras, and watches.

"You can see there's plenty of money around Tingo," observed Ramon.

At the restaurant we dispatched a few hot dogs and drank Coca Cola, to avoid the germ-infested local water. On our way back to the monastery, Jean-Michel appeared thoughtful. In the vast starry canopy the Southern Cross shone over us.

"I'm thinking," he said, "of all the victims of cocaine, those thousands of miles away, who look for a high and a kick, and those right here caught trying to escape their misery. They don't know about each other, but they're exploited by the same drug mafia."

He added, "We'll have a better idea of the dimensions of the problem after tomorrow's trip. The Peruvian police are taking us on a mission to destroy an illegal coca plantation."

23

The Traffickers of Juan Juy

The next day at dawn a spanking new twin-engine plane picked us up at the end of the deserted runway of the Tingo Maria airport. We flew over the Huallaga River, one of the waterways of the Amazon High Valley, winding through the thick green jungle. On each side of the river the forest stretched as far as the eye could see, impenetrable, with no visible traces of human presence, but dotted here and there with small lighter patches.

"Coca plantations," Captain Ramon told us.

He also pointed to an oil palm plantation partly nestled in the wide curve of the river, covering thousands of acres with perfectly aligned rows of trees in sharp contrast with the surrounding chaotic vegetation. At the center of the plantation a factory and its tall brick stack reminded the traveler of the civilized world.

"In this valley," added Ramon, "enough fruit and vegetables could be grown to feed all of South America."

A storm blew out of the sky, unexpectedly. Our small plane was pitched and tossed by the elements. There was no visibility through the rain–drenched windows. If we hadn't been strapped to our seats, we would have been thrown across the cabin. The smiling pilot, clutching his levers, would glance from time to time at the picture of a well–endowed señorita in a swim suit strumming her mandoline and covering the radar screen.

The sun reappeared as quickly as it had disappeared, and Ramon pointed out a long runway built in the heart of the jungle.

"On that runway, planes like this one land regularly to

pick up the coca paste and fly it to Colombia, about two hundred miles north. It's a concrete runway, very difficult to destroy. The planes land and take off in fifteen minutes, just long enough to load their cargo of paste and drop off the chemicals used to make it. To intercept them we'd have to be on location when they land. Since we don't have any planes to bring us over, we'd have to come up the river by boat and then walk five or six hours through the jungle."

The plane started its descent towards a large clearing where a few low houses lined the river.

"That's Juan Juy," said Ramon.

The pilot flew over a herd of cows that dispersed, frightened by the noise. The plane regained altitude and circled the village before landing on a dirt runway invaded by grass, under the eyes of the peaceful bovines who had hastily yielded part of their territory.

Near a wooden hut on the edge of the meadow a police detachment invited us to climb into their four-wheel drive dusty vans. "They're going to show us how they destroy an illegal coca plantation located twenty-five miles, as the crow flies, from Juan Juy," said Jean-Michel.

Ignoring the potholes of the dirt road, the vans raced along and we could barely hold on to our seats.

At the first crossroad, near a soldiers' outpost, several police agents clustered around a pickup truck and were waving their machine guns. We stopped our vans and saw the traffickers they had arrested. A man, about eighteen, was grabbed by the hair and hit with the rifle butts while one of the agents brandished bags full of coca paste.

"He was carrying four pounds," he exclaimed.

"What's the sentence for that?" asked Jean-Michel.

"At least fifteen years."

We started off, a little more slowly this time. The condition of the road, frequently gouged by trenches cut by torrential rains, slowed our speed to a walking rate.

"In tropical climates like ours, it's impossible to maintain good roads," Jeri explained. "It rains too much and the earth crumbles. It would take tons of rock and concrete to build a road bed. That's one reason we have so much trouble developing the region in spite of its rich soil."

The vans were periodically stopped by weighted poles

blocking the road near crudely-assembled wooden huts that sheltered the police agents. A few words were exchanged between them and the P.P.F. forces, and we would lumber on.

"This region is sparsely populated," Jeri told us. "We have nothing to fear around here. However, some three hundred miles south, near Ayacucho, it gets more dangerous because the guerilla soldiers of the "Shining Path"[1] control a good part of the province."

The road stopped suddenly in the middle of the jungle and our little troop, surrounded by a force of half a dozen police, alighted. The "delinquent" farmer, fiftyish, with a goatee, hollow cheeks, and frightened eyes, walked in his bare feet, taking the lead through grassy plots intermingled with small trees and dense hedges. The moist, stifling heat made the climb difficult, especially for Jean-Paul Cornu weighted down with his camera equipment and Guy Jouas with his sound equipment.

The police carried cans of insecticide and a spray gun, in addition to their firearms. We were walking at a good pace, leaving the meadows behind us and climbing through the forest along a path furrowed by torrents that we crossed knee-deep in muddy water.

Suddenly the column came to a standstill. I welcomed the pause and sank to the ground, exhausted. Our guide had spied a wire stretched across the path. He must have had keen eyesight, because we were moving in the dusky penumbra of a thick underbrush. Suddenly, a shot rang out. I leaped to my feet in a flash, ready to take off. But I heard laughter and guffaws. Dominique Simian, one of the explorers with the Cousteau expedition, and a police agent were defusing an explosive contraption rigged with a sawed-off shotgun. The police told us the explosive was probably placed there to protect a clandestine coca paste lab.

"Do you realize what that can do to you?" asked Simian.

"Blow off your leg," said Jean-Michel, shaking his head.

We now followed a path leading to a stream that leaped noisily in the underbrush. We reached the well-hidden "laboratory" poised on the edge of the water. Coca leaves were soaking in a tub-shaped hole dug in the ground and covered with a black plastic sheet fixed with wooden pegs.

"What's that mixture?" asked Jean-Michel.

"Water with sulfuric acid, kerosene, and bicarbonate of

soda," answered Jeri. "The plastic containers that come full of chemicals are used when empty to carry water from the stream and for the preparation of the paste."

The police poured gasoline over the soaking foliage and set it on fire after emptying a few bags of coca leaves they had discovered nearby. A thick black smoke billowed up, exuding an acrid, unbearable odor. I held my breath.

"Watch out," smiled Jeri. "You inhale three puffs of that smoke and you'll find yourself on a cloud."

As we resumed our trek, Jeri explained that there are thousands of such labs scattered through the countryside, providing tidy profits for the farmers. To twenty-five pounds of leaves worth about five dollars, the farmer adds chemicals that cost him twenty dollars. The dried concoction yields about forty grams of paste that is sold for forty dollars to a dealer. Three batches of paste a week will clear a forty-five dollar profit and bring him one hundred and eighty dollars a month.

"It isn't much."

"For the farmer it's plenty, ten times more than a crop of bananas or guavas."

We paused to chew pieces of sugar cane stalk that a police agent cut down on the side of the path. The juice of the plant was delicious and quenched our thirst.

At last we reached the illegal coca plantation: a little over an acre of coca trees growing on the stripped slope of the mountain.

The old man's first gesture was to pick a few leaves that he put in his toothless mouth and started to chew slowly. His face, like the face of any coca chewer, was a blank.

Jeri asked him, for Jean-Michel, if he knew he was risking a fifteen-year jail sentence for illegally growing coca bushes. The man didn't appear to understand what we were saying and looked at us with a stunned expression.

"I'm not guilty of anything," he finally said. "I planted these bushes for my own use. I've always chewed coca leaves."

"And the lab we found down there?"

"I've never seen it before."

In the meanwhile, a police agent wearing a gas mask sprayed the coca bushes with herbicide he had brought along.

It was improbable that the farmer had never seen the laboratory, but he certainly had not recently prepared coca paste: his fingers were not swollen around the nails, nor yellowed, nor corroded by the acid concoction in which the coca leaves are soaked. The old man witnessed with disbelief the destruction of his coca field. He shook his head.

We turned around to leave. The climb down was difficult because we kept slipping on the water-logged clay. Our group stopped near a large hut with a thatched roof. It was the "delinquent's" farm. His wife, an aged woman, white-haired and stooped, who had seen us go by on our way up, invited us to eat. She had prepared a chicken stew with plantains.

Never had I seen such a miserable, run-down farm. The yard was a stinking mud-hole where pigs wallowed. The shack had a single large room with a dirt floor and one window. The only furniture was a table and a bench.

I was famished. I swallowed some thin broth from a chipped bowl, then walked with Jeri towards the meadow to escape the nauseating stench in the courtyard. We noticed orange trees that yielded small green oranges, stringy and tasteless.

"All the oranges are like that around here," said Jeri. "Plenty of fruit trees could be grown in this region, but the farmers don't know how to care for them and they're too poor to invest in the products needed for productive cultivation. These slopes could be covered by beautiful orchards."

A police agent set a pail full of murky smelly water in front of us.

The men drank directly from it. I was tempted to do the same and looked at Jeri for advice.

"Better not," he said. "This water is contaminated, like all the streams around here, with everything you can think of: amoebae, flukes, schistosomes — all sorts of parasites that cause abscesses of the liver and the brain.

We returned by a different route and at nightfall reached a small town. Its white stuccoed belfrey glowed in the setting sun. Seated around the only table in the village inn, we drank with relish a few bottles of Coke. Once in a while a customer would stroll in to buy a cigarette or two, sold piecemeal from a pack. There wasn't much else for sale in the store, except toilet paper and soft drinks. Behind the counter, a young woman smoked a cigarette next to a small boy whose head I could barely see. I was intrigued by the smoke that seemed to curl out of the child's hair. I walked over and saw the boy puffing away, slowly exhaling the smoke through his nose.

"How old is this little fellow?" I asked.

"Four," she answered, somewhat embarrassed. "I know he shouldn't be smoking, he's too young. But if I don't give him a cigarette, he starts crying."

We arrived at Juan Juy too late to take the plane back to Tingo Maria. The pilot, who refused to navigate on instruments, had no ground communications and never flew after sunset. We were forced to spend the night in Juan Juy's only hotel. I was so tired that, oblivious to the filth of the room, I dropped on a lumpy mattress. I was jolted out of a deep sleep a few hours later by gunshots. Shouts and jeers promptly relieved my fears. A fiesta or a wedding must have been in progress. But sleep eluded me, and I began to think about the past day.

Going through this trying expedition just to witness the destruction of an acre and a half of coca seemed an exercise in futility. I wasn't sorry I had come, however. Now I had a better perspective on the dimensions of the problem of coca–growing in Peru. The economy of the country is in such a state of disarray that the cultivation of the coca bush represents the only way for the farmer to escape his destitute condition. Paradoxically, he is in no position to develop the natural resources of a rich land, to grow the fruit, the cereals, or the vegetables or to raise the cattle he and his family need so badly.

With no professional training, isolated from the modern world, in the midst of a barebones economic system, the Peruvian farmer lives in poverty. He sees in the coca trade the only way to make a little money. He doesn't suspect that the poison extracted from coca leaves will kill other men, well-fed and well-housed, in an unknown distant country.

On the other hand, the methods used by the Peruvian authorities to destroy a few illegal patches of coca trees seemed farcical. Even the spraying of herbicides by helicopters over large areas, as Colonel Vargas suggested, appears impractical in view of the widely scattered locations of the crops. Herbicides don't discriminate between good and bad plants, and in any event the bad plants eventually grow back. These methods of eradication prove much too costly even for the United States. Moreover, the guerillas would take an evil pleasure in destroying the helicopters with their missiles.

What about the phyloxera? I thought. At the beginning of the century that voracious insect devoured the roots of grapevines and in a few years destroyed all the vineyards in France. An antidote came from the United States in the form of a hardy California vine that resisted the parasite's teeth and thus starved it to death. More recently a small mushroom has been killing most of the elms in the United States and Europe by choking their sap capillaries, and no antidote has been found to stop the devastation. To eradicate the coca tree, a natural plague would be sufficient. Such a plague has not sprung up yet, but modern science could create one. A plant geneticist could easily assemble a virus that would become the deadly parasite of the plant genome, the part that contains the genetic code of the species. This type of virus has a high specificity and will only attack the species for which it is designed. Similar specific viruses already exist in nature, such as the mosaic virus of tobacco. Once the virus is created, it has to be promptly disseminated. For that, natural carriers could be used: the wind would blow the contaminated dead leaves. Insects might help do the job. An entomologist could load viruses into the winged insects which naturally lodge in the coca bush and transform them into carriers that would propagate the pest throughout the plantation. If we could do with the coca bush what the Dutch Elm disease did to the elms, it would be a good start.

The next morning, I shared my thoughts with Jeri. He shook his head.

"You had nightmares last night."

Then he added, as an afterthought, "You know, my friend, it might not be such a crazy idea, but not today or even tomorrow. Maybe later, much, much later."

On the bumpy flight back to Tingo Maria I sighted many illicit light green plantations of coca dotting the dark jungle. While realizing how difficult it would be to implement an eradication program, I remained convinced that it was the only solution to control the illicit cocaine traffic. I was reminded of the analogy between external and internal pollution which was foremost in Captain Cousteau's mind when he organized our expedition into the sources of cocaine production. Once an industrial plant has released its toxic wastes into the environment, it is too late to protect the surrounding population, and one can only limit the extent of the damage caused by the contamination. When cocaine has reached its prosperous foreign markets, it spreads like an epidemic and only a small portion of the drug is seized and destroyed. The motto of the Cousteau Society, "To protect the environment from pollutants through advanced technology," could also be applied to the control of the cocaine epidemic at its source.

As we droned along, I daydreamed that methods used currently in biotechnology were available for coca bush eradication and they were ecologically sound, but their implementation could not be carried out at the present time by the Peruvian government even with the help of the United States. A long-term international assistance program was required, which would couple coca bush eradication with the growing of basic food crops in the fertile valleys and fruit trees on the gentle slopes. The illiterate farmers would be educated and learn modern agricultural techniques and farm management. Tractors would replace hoes, paved roads would run through the countryside. Cattle would graze in the meadows. I thought of the Marshall plan which contributed so decisively to the rebuilding of western Europe after the Second World War. A similar plan for Peru was not for today, as Raoul Jeri had concluded. Indeed, such a plan, in order to be successful, would have to enlist the unanimous support and cooperation of the medical establishment in the Americas. And this was not the case either in North or South America, as our visit with Dr. Cabieses and with the officials of E.N.A.C.O. had so clearly revealed. As long as the redeeming value of the coca leaf is recognized, how can one eradicate the coca bush?

A sudden violent jolt interrupted my dreams as our plane flew through turbulent air pockets. I returned to reality as we were about to land in Tingo Maria.

V

TO WIN THE COCAINE WARS:
A BATTLE OF THE MINDS

24

Consuming and Producing Countries: Shared Responsibilities

After our return to Lima, Jean-Michel had an audience with the president of the Republic of Peru, Fernando Belaunde, and later the same night he joined us for dinner at the Hotel Bolivar. For the first time since the beginning of his Amazonian expedition, he was wearing a suit and tie. He seemed even more thoughtful than usual, while telling about his meeting with the president.

"Belaunde is a very distinguished and educated gentleman. After a long and difficult struggle he was instrumental in reinstating a parliamentary democracy in Peru. However, he refuses to assume any responsibility for the cocaine problem. He didn't mince his words. 'We, in Peru, are very grateful for what western society has brought us in the areas of arts, literature, technology, medicine, and many others. But we owe you no gratitude for the traffic of cocaine which is a foreign enterprise. I am convinced that this problem is the responsibility of the consumer countries rather than the producing countries.' "

I felt that President Belaunde was simplifying the problem. The growing demand generated by the United States contributed to an increase in the traffic. However, the underdeveloped economic conditions prevailing in Peru have equally favored the growth of an illegal trade which, in fact, results from the converging interests of two societies at a critical stage of their history. On one side, the underdeveloped economy of the coca-producing Peruvian jungle coupled with widespread poverty is breeding corruption; and on the other side, the affluent American consumer society and its hedonistic wastefulness leads to the recreational use of drugs.

However, it would be unfair to lay all the responsibility for cocaine traffic at the door of the United States, which owes its remarkable development and its power to a culture fundamentally opposed to recreational drug use. Its laws, repressive on that issue, are attempting to curb the cocaine epidemic. Rather, it would be better to determine each side's responsibilities, not to judge either party but to attempt an assessment of the problem in its broadest dimension.

It seems clear that the extensive recreational use of cocaine was preceded in the United States by the social acceptance of drug intoxication and, in recent years, by the erosion of a taboo that banned the consumption of illicit drugs. The reversal of moral values that held to the age-old tenet of "a healthy mind in a healthy body" first appeared in the most prestigious American universities, and peaked with the student revolts in the late sixties. Like many others, I was witness to this cultural revolution of freedom without restraints that counted among its leaders Timothy Leary, Herbert Marcuse, and Aldous Huxley, followed by a host of specialists in psychiatry and the social sciences. The momentum was such that even many churches yielded and adjusted to the new provisional ethics of a liberated society. As for scientists, and more specifically molecular biologists, frequently isolated in the ivory tower of their computerized laboratories, they often lacked perspective and were unable to stem the cultural tidal wave.

Many psychopharmacologists restrict their studies of the brain to a few biochemical reactions which occur on isolated fragments. If such painstaking investigations are essential for a better understanding of one of the many mechanisms involved in cerebral activity, they tend to detach the scientists from a broader perspective of overall function of the whole organ. As one of these scientists confided to me: "What can I tell you about cocaine-related brain toxicity? My area of specialization is the passage of calcium through channels of the cellular membrane."

Could a detached attitude of this kind be explained by the climate of uncertainty born from the cultural revolution which eroded the moral imperatives that guided scientists like Louis Pasteur or Ludwig Lewin a century ago?

In the light of the collective resignation of their intellectual mentors, millions of youth adopted the naive libertarian ideas of bygone years, reformulated by brilliant but misguided

intellectuals and amplified by the media. In the name of freedom, young people became the victims—unwittingly yet enthusiastically—of slogans extolling the right to pleasure and to
a chemically-induced mystical experience.

The Peruvian authorities find themselves in an ambiguous position, accepting the consumption of the coca leaf but
banning that of cocaine. Since Peru regained its independence
a century and a half ago, the government has continued to
grant the Indians the right to chew coca leaves, while underestimating the harmful effects of the habit on their health. At
the same time, the recreational use of cocaine was always
sternly condemned by Peruvian society. All this was clearly
explained to us during the Cousteau expedition by Dr. Cabieses and the bureaucrats who manage E.N.A.C.O. This ambiguity became even more apparent to me, a year later, when I
delivered a lecture on the toxicology of cocaine at the School of
Medicine of San Marcos in Lima. At the end of my talk,
several of my Peruvian colleagues expressed their surprise,
because I had insisted on the harmful effects of cocaine while
omitting the benefits of its moderate use "recommended by
certain American scholars from Harvard." A professor of pharmacology at San Marcos University mentioned the hypo-
glycemic effect of an extract of coca leaves, which he himself
had studied, and he handed me a handsome brochure in English, published by the The Beneficial Plant Research Association.[1]

This association, founded in the United States in 1979[2] to
study and promote the use of plants which will improve the
quality of human life, was headed by a botanist, Timothy
Plowman, and the physician Andrew Weil, both from Harvard. The members of the Association's scientific advisory
board included two personalities mentioned earlier: Dr.
Ronald Siegel of Los Angeles and Dr. Fernando Cabieses of
Lima. The roster also included Drs. Lester Grinspoon and
Norman Zinberg of Harvard, both psychiatrists and advocates
of the legalization of marijuana, and well-known scientists such
as the Swiss chemist Albert Hofman who discovered L.S.D.,
the Stockholm toxicologist Bo Holmstedt, and botanists William Evans from Nottingham and Richard Evans Schultes
from Harvard.

One of the articles in the Association's brochure mentions
the beneficial effects of cocaine leaves on Peruvian Indians to

justify one of its chief objectives: the development of a coca-leaf "natural" extract to be used in common pharmaceutical preparations such as syrups, tablets, gumdrops, or potions. The multiple medical uses suggested by the Association members were reminiscent of those listed a hundred years ago by Freud in *Uber Coca:* as a remedy for gastritis, stomach ulcers and laryngitis, for weight reduction and as a quick-acting antidepressant.

The Association had even devised new therapeutic applications for the ancient cocaine extract: "a substitute for coffee in patients unable to tolerate it, a cure against sea-sickness, a regulator of sugar metabolism in diabetes and hypoglycemia."

No one questions the good intentions of these scientists, but one may wonder at their näiveté, lack of pharmacological knowledge, and ignorance of history. Since the end of World War II, researchers have enriched our modern pharmacopeia with specific and effective remedies to treat the ailments allegedly cured by coca leaf extracts; and this is achieved without inducing dependency since strict regulations, spelled out in the Harrison Act of 1914, forbid the commercial availability of any cocaine–containing medication.

Historical observations, in ancient and modern times, have established that the coca alkaloid is the most habit-forming substance in the plant world. Lewin plainly describes its properties: "One starts with small amounts and one keeps increasing them to reach daily intoxicating doses."

Therefore the use of coca leaf extract as recommended by the Beneficial Plant Research Association is in no way medically justified and should have been rebutted by more knowledgeable pharmacologists or physicians. Nothing of the kind happened, as if the authors of the recommendations were too renowned to be challenged. Consequently, the Association's declarations provided the Peruvian authorities with new arguments to justify the acceptance of the coca leaf chewing by the Andean populations.

The responsibility of American and European intellectuals, influenced by the cultural revolution of the sixties, which promulgated the moderate "recreational" use of cocaine, becomes now only too apparent: besides encouraging the social acceptance of the drug in the western world, their endorsements justified the continued cultivation and consumption of coca in the producing countries. Opinion makers of today are all the more responsible since their assumptions about Indians chewing coca leaves for beneficial purposes are not scientifically acceptable.

Indeed, as Dr. Fernandez told us, all medical studies of Andean populations have concluded that the consumption of coca leaves damages the mental and physical health of the Indians. Professor Albert Buck, a Johns Hopkins epidemiologist, published, in 1968, a well documented study in the *American Journal of Epidemiology*.[3] Buck compares the health of abstemious Indians with the health of coca leaf chewers, both from the Peruvian village of Cachicoto. The coca chewers suffer from malnutrition and are underweight; in addition their albumin and cholesterol blood concentrations are inferior to those of abstemious Indians. Malnutrition seriously affects chewers suffering from anemia caused by intestinal parasites. Anemia is less severe among those with better eating habits. Infections and infectious diseases, which cause a weakening of the immune system and consequently lead to a higher absenteeism at the workplace, are more widespread among coca chewers than among abstemious subjects.

Buck attributes those deficiencies to the indirect effects of coca which maintain the users in a continuous state of malnutrition traceable to a decrease in the sensations of hunger and fatigue, caused by the coca alkaloid. These observations confirm the experimental studies which indicate that cocaine alters the brain areas that control activities closely related to survival, such as thirst and hunger.

Dr. Juan Negrete,[4] from McGill University, compared the intellectual faculties of coca-chewing farmers and those of abstemious subjects in a small village in northern Argentina. In this study, published in 1967 in the *Narcotics Bulletin* of the United Nations, Negrete reports that coca users display loss of memory and attention span, and that their intellectual performances are lower than those of the abstemious subjects.

Finally, it is now established that coca leaf chewers consume daily thirty to sixty grams of coca leaves containing 200 to 500 milligrams of cocaine, which clearly is an intoxicating dose. It is four to ten times larger than the fifty to one hundred milligrams swallowed in a little water by Freud and which endowed him with self control and euphoria while dissipating hunger and fatigue.

Furthermore, a group of American scientists from Yale University measured the blood levels of native coca leaf chewers and reported "pharmacologically significant concentrations similar to those presented by American recreational snorters of the drug."

Scientific research therefore supports, nearly one hundred years later, Lewin's conclusions about the harmful effects of coca chewing on the physical and mental health of the Indians, conclusions based upon his interpretation of history and his training as a physiologist and a physician.

Buck and Negrete's studies were conducted in the sixties with the support of the United Nations in an effort to document the harmful effects of cocaine use in developing countries. But these studies received little or no attention because at that same time a cultural revolution was challenging the standards upheld throughout a fifty-year struggle to contain the spread of cocaine and habit-forming drugs. One of the spokesmen of this new culture was a Washington social anthropologist, Dr. William Carter, who, in the late seventies, undertook a study of Indian farmers and mine workers in Bolivia. He reported that ninety-five percent of them chewed coca leaves daily "and were in good health." He then concluded: "To ban the use of coca among Indians in the name of our western values would be tantamount to committing a new ethnocide."[5] Nowadays, many intellectuals prefer to ignore the scientific conclusions of Buck and Negrete and to embrace the hypothesis of Freud as reworded by William Carter and the Association for Research on Beneficial Plants.

In such a climate of ambiguity, Peru is powerless to develop effective measures to curb cocaine traffic, which would first require a rigorous control of the cultivation of the coca bush. The government appears equally unable to consider the gradual limitation of the use of the coca leaf by the Andean population, a challenging task which would necessarily entail a program of social and economic development to allow the integration of the Indian population into the mainstream of Peruvian society. Such a project would call for a national consensus along with help from the international community and a cultural and social policy of rejection of the use of coca.

One should note that most of the Indians who do not chew coca leaves are *evangelicos,* Evangelical Protestants.[6] They embrace a religion where the use of coca is taboo, incompatible with the practice of the Christian faith. This observation, reported by both Buck and Carter in Peru and Bolivia, illustrates the importance of the cultural milieu in the rejection of drug use. Since a massive religious conversion of the Indian population is improbable in the 20th century, another motivation will have to be found to orient them towards a drug-free life.

If, as its leaders claim, the United States wants to set itself before the world as an example of a model society, its responsibility for controlling the cocaine trade looms larger than that of Peru. Unfortunately the image of the United States projected abroad is that of a drug–consuming nation. Its capacity to wage an effective fight against cocaine consumption has been hampered by intellectuals who condone the recreational use of drugs and claim to do so in the name of the great American ideals of freedom and human rights.

The cultural mutation in the United States remains the principal cause of the social acceptance of recreational drug use which has become so prevalent throughout the country. Very few voices from academia have risen to resist this new trend, however opposed the silent majority might be to the few iconoclasts and pied pipers who profess to free the human mind from its demons and Prometheus from his chains. The 20th Century followers of the old libertarian sophists have enjoyed a free hand to accomplish their demolition task with extraordinary ease and speed. The general acceptance of their theses resulted, within twenty years, in an unprecedented disaster for western society.

However, the revolutionaries of the sixties failed to suggest an alternative route to the rising generations lured by their enticing slogans: "To forbid is forbidden" and "To moralize is immoral." At the same time they remained somewhat respectful of science which became, for the modern world, the great fountain of truth.

And today, science, and more precisely the life sciences, should provide the compelling principles around which the western mind can rally to ensure its survival in tomorrow's world. Indeed the lesson is clear: in any society, from the most technologically advanced to the most underdeveloped, the trivialization of drug use leads to human degradation and social decline. It is time for intellectuals in the west to redefine the values that chart the social progress of a civilization, and to subscribe, if it is not already too late, to the international agreements that ban the use of the most destructive drugs of dependence, except for medical and scientific investigations.

25

The Cold War and the Business of Cocaine

In the course of its forays into the Colombian jungle of the Upper Valley of the Amazon, Captain Cousteau's team made contact with a young teacher of mathematics turned leader of a band of guerilleros. We will call him "Lopez." Several of his meetings with Jean-Michel were filmed. He is seen in the videofilm, *Snowstorm in the Jungle,*[1] with his face hidden from the cameras to protect his anonymity.

Lopez acknowledged right away that cultivation and illegal traffic of drugs are widely spread in the area where his group operates.

"All the local population is involved," he told us, "farmers, merchants, police agents. The bishop is the only clean one!" He admitted that his own men have a hand in this lucrative business.

"Do you know," Jean-Michel asked, "that in the United States young people consume cocaine extracted from leaves or coca paste and that some of them die?"

"In Latin America," answered Lopez, "the number of victims of North American imperialism is huge. So why should we be shocked when cocaine kills a few people in the United States?" He spoke without bitterness, with a hint of irony in his voice as if he were discussing a casual deal. He was voicing the popular resentment against the Giant of the North and justifying the collusion between guerrillas of the revolution and the drug traffickers. Coca is, indeed, an exchange currency for the purchase of arms shipped through illicit and secret routes, the same as those used by the drug trade.

It is clear that cocaine contributes indirectly to the political destabilization of the governments of Peru and Colombia, democratically elected but nevertheless fragile. The role played by the Marxist governments of Cuba and Nicaragua in the combined traffic of cocaine sent to the United States and armaments shipped to the guerilleros is difficult to document. This dual traffic is run by secret services one of whose prime concerns is to cover up their tracks. Proof of collusion surfaces in confessions of turncoat agents and reports leaked by North American intelligence agencies.

There is no doubt that guerrilla armaments coming from the Communist bloc countries do not reach their South American destinations through regular commercial channels. For years these arms have been fueling an actual civil war, spearheaded in Colombia by the M-14 movement and in Peru by the militants of the "Shining Path" or the "Tupac Amaru." On both sides, guerilla and government forces, the victims add up to thousands, not counting losses among unfortunate civilian populations caught in the cross-fire.

The Marxist regimes that support armed insurrections in South America vehemently deny any involvement in drug traffic, which they view as an enterprise entirely managed by the "corrupt plutocracy of capitalist countries." It must be noted that in the social rules imposed on their own citizenry, the people's republics have reclaimed many of the moral principles on which parliamentarian democracies were built. Drug use is considered a highly antisocial practice and is punished by death. Cocaine or opiate addictions have not taken root in the USSR which follows a policy of strict punishment of drug addicts and vigilant efforts to suppress drug supplies. Cuba is the only land in the American hemisphere where drug consumption is not widely spread.

The Kremlin leaders and their allies face a powerful adversary with whom they have been locked until now in a struggle for the control of the planet. They are aware of the stakes and are likely to take advantage of the weaknesses of their opponent and its Achilles' heel, all the more so since drug and arms traffic is cloaked in secrecy and uses several intermediaries, making it impossible to incriminate the Soviets directly. In addition, the operation is highly profitable since it is financed by their adversary. The major drug dealers pay cash for the shipping of cocaine to its final destination and the money is used for the purchase of armaments which go to the guerillas scattered in coca growing areas. The political benefits of this cold war operation are enormous since the United States will be hurt at home and abroad. Abroad, governments allied to the United States are weakened by guerillas plotting their overthrow. At home, cocaine contributes to the corruption of the American capitalist system which is in fact financing its own downfall. Machiavelli[2] couldn't have plotted a subtler device to destroy a powerful enemy.

Drug enforcement and intelligence agencies of the United States have several times implicated the Republic of Cuba in the traffic of cocaine into the United States and of arms in support of South American guerilla forces. The large island of Cuba, located five hundred miles from Colombia and only ninety miles from Florida, has a privileged geographic position as a logistic stepping stone between North and South America in the arms-for-cocaine trade, both by air and by sea. Hundreds of neighboring islands in the Caribbean Sea, some of them deserted, can provide additional ports of call. Moreover, the United States has no diplomatic or commercial ties with Cuba, whose economic survival depends wholly on the Soviet bloc. Americans can hardly afford to pressure their small neighbor and its leader, Fidel Castro, without triggering an international incident.

The role played by the Cuban authorities in arms and cocaine traffic has been studied in great detail in numerous testimonies received in Miami in May, 1983, by the Senate committee[3] in charge of drug control and presided over by the then Florida Senator, Paula Hawkins.[4] According to Cuban defectors–turned–informants, such as Mario Estebes Gonzales, Gerardo Peraza and David Perez, the Cuban government, more precisely the Central Committee of the Cuban Communist Party, headed by Fidel Castro, decided in 1979 to participate actively in the logistics of cocaine trade as it related to arms traffic. Cuba's role began in the fall of 1980 when one hundred and twenty-five thousand Cubans were shipped to the United States with the agreement of the American authorities in the course of "Operation Mariel."[5] The majority of the Cubans were political prisoners whose families had recently settled in Florida. But these "politicals" were accompanied by several thousand common criminals — Castro had taken the opportunity to empty his jails — and three thousand Cuban secret service agents. Those agents had been especially trained to organize cocaine distribution networks in Florida and North America. One of them, Mario Estebes Gonzales, a defector, provided the data.

The Hawkins Committee states that the Cuban role in cocaine traffic was officially condemned by American authorities in the fall of 1982. At that time, the Florida Attorney General, Stanley Marcus, indicted in absentia four high officials of the Republic of Cuba, members of the Communist Party Central Committee, for their role in a "communist conspiracy related to drug trafficking." The individuals charged were Rene Rodriguez Cruz, one of the heads of the Cuban Information Services who organized the transfer of the hundred and twenty-five thousand Cubans who came to Florida under Operation Mariel in 1980; Admiral Aldo Santamaria-Cuadrado, accused of organizing the shipments of cocaine by boat from Colombia to Florida via Cuba; Fernando Ravelo-Rencido, an ambassador of Cuba to Colombia; and Gonzalo Bossols Suarez, a former Cuban ambassador. The last two were accused of organizing cocaine traffic networks in Colombia with the help of a Colombian shipbuilder, Jaime Gillot-Lara. They were expelled from Colombia when it broke diplomatic relations with Cuba in 1981. The indictment was "conspiracy at the highest levels to organize the traffic of cocaine between South American producers and North American consumers." This organization established a complex network that began with the cultivation of the coca bush and the preparation of the coca paste, continued with delivery to clandestine laboratories in Colombia to refine the paste into powder, and finally shipped the cargo through various intermediaries, by air or sea, to Cuba. With the complicity of Cuban agents and crews, the drug was introduced into Florida where large dealers supplied small retailers who then channelled it to distribution points around the United States.

These successive steps are described in detail in testimony by former Cuban secret agents turned informers after their capture by American agents on planes or ships carrying cocaine or armaments. The Cuban high officials, assumed leaders of the small agents, were accused by American authorities of master-minding the drug trafficking but never appeared before the Miami tribunal. The agent Esteves, who was granted a suspended sentence, declared that the Cuban government has asked him to ship, via Cuba, five hundred kilos of cocaine a month. He claimed that the Cuban authorities set the price of cocaine for the Colombian trader at fifty thousand dollars per kilo, on which they slapped a ten percent tax, thus milking a two and a half million dollar profit a month for Cuba, no negligible sum for a country starved for hard currency. Esteves also claimed that the Cuban Navy helped the illegal cargo ships in avoiding detection by American coast-guard radar.

These sensational revelations contained in Paula Hawkins' Senate Commission Report received official clearance and were widely publicized in the media. The Cuban defectors appeared on all the major T.V. networks, and their testimony was reproduced in detail in the press. A month after the Hawkins Committee Hearings, President Reagan declared:

> We have the proof that officials of the Castro regime are implicated in drug traffic which makes them criminals exploiting the misery of the addicts. I wish to seize this opportunity to appeal to the Castro regime to be accountable for its actions. Is this traffic carried out by corrupt officials or is it carried out with the official knowledge of Castro? The world demands an answer.

In rather undiplomatic language Reagan was asking a direct question. Castro's answer was a harsh denial: "Untruthful allegations meant to conceal the responsibilities of American imperialism," he retorted.

This indictment of Cuba's role in the flow of cocaine to the United States led nowhere. The racial riots in South Africa and the Middle-East conflict once more dominated the daily news while at the same time cocaine traffic, in spite of increased seizures, continued to grow. Since 1983, the white powder has been entering the United States, with or without Cuban help, in ever-increasing amounts, through the Caribbean Sea, which remains the major transit route between Colombia and the United States. The West Indies are beginning to be seriously affected, especially the Bahaman islands which are the closest to the Colombian shores.[6]

In the Spring of 1986 I was invited by Dr. Timothy McCartney, who directs a drug rehabilitation center in Nassau, the capitol of the Bahamas. I was appalled by the extent of cocaine addiction on that island which, with a population of a little over one hundred thousand, numbers several thousands of coca paste or "crack" smokers. In the two Nassau psychiatric hospitals there were no admissions for cocaine psychosis in 1982. In 1983 there were sixty-nine, in 1984 five hundred and twenty-three. The authorities are powerless to curb the disaster. Dr. McCartney told me about a macabre ritual performed by young addicts in this paradise island. The game is known as the Return from Yonder. Two or three cocaine addicts train themselves in life-saving methods to treat respiratory or cardiac arrest. They proceed to smoke "crack" until one of them passes out and appears dead. The survivors then attempt to resuscitate the victim and bring him back from his trip into the other world, without always succeeding.

In South America the guerilla movement continues, especially in the Peruvian and Colombian jungles where coca is grown or processed. If Cuba has not recently been incriminated in the cocaine traffic, Nicaragua has been directly accused several times by the American authorities. The Marxist-leaning Sandinista government as well as the CIA–supported Contras have both been implicated.[7]

It appears that the cocaine traffic which might have been initially supported by leftist political interventions has now become an independent well-managed business enterprise fueled by the massive profits it has generated. Big money has the power to corrupt political figures whatever their ideological political convictions may be. The indictment by the United States Justice Department of General Manuel Antonio Noriega,[8] head of the Armed Forces of Panama, for his involvement in the cocaine traffic is a case in point. More than two years after his indictment, the General is still Commander–in–Chief in his country and defying his mighty neighbor. One wonders how he has been able to remain in power in spite of the economic sanctions enforced by the United States against Panama.

Another political figure who has been implicated but never indicted in the cocaine trade is the popular Prime Minister of the Bahamas, Lynden Pindling. While the many casinos and the offshore banks of Nassau are ideal places to launder the tainted drug money, the dozens of islands of the Bahamian archipelago, such as Norman Kay, provide excellent, well-concealed trans-shipment points between the Colombian coastline and Florida. All of the alleged dealings of the Colombia warlords and their underlings with the Noriegas and the Pindlings have been described in *The Cocaine Wars,* a book published by three intrepid journalists, Paul Eddy, Hugo Sabogal, and Sara Walden.[9]

I became aware of the power of cocaine traffickers during a lecture tour of Peru and Colombia organized by the United States Information Agency of the State Department in February 1984. It was a long harassing trip and my wife paid her own way to be at my side. We were assigned a bodyguard and were driven in a bullet-proof car in Bogota and in Medellin, the world center of the cocaine traffic. Each time our car stopped at a red light, our bodyguard scrutinized the adjoining cars and motorcycles, ready to pull his gun.

In the course of my visit I had the opportunity to meet the Colombian Minister of Justice, Lara Bonila, who had undertaken to fight the drug lords. He assured me he was going to pursue his task to the end, despite the threats he had received. Two months later I learned he had been shot by a motorcyclist when his car stopped at a light. The killer admitted he had received twenty thousand dollars from the drug mafia to do the job.

At the end of his film *Snowstorm on the Jungle,* Captain Cousteau, referring to the Opium War of a hundred years ago in Asia, declares: "Today the Americas are the theatre of a cocaine war." In the new merciless war that is ravaging the Americas, Cuba, the only country which has been able to maintain a taboo against the use of cocaine, could play a determining role. If the United States wants to fight drug traffic efficiently at its source, the cooperation of Cuba could be invaluable. But are the Americans ready to change their South American policy?

Nonetheless, the traffic of cocaine is entirely financed by the American consumers who disburse extravagant sums to satisfy their craving for the drug. *The Financial Times* of May 24, 1985, estimates that a kilo of cocaine sold wholesale for eight thousand dollars in Bogotá will reach thirty thousand dollars (some say fifty thousand) when it arrives in the United States, before it is retailed! The quantity exported is of the order of two hundred thousand kilos per year, ten to twenty percent of which is seized or lost en route. The traffic therefore generates a revenue of five billion dollars for the producing countries of South America. In the United States, the prices escalate as the drug trickles down to the consumers. The retail value of a kilo of cocaine, which has lost a half or a quarter of its pure drug content, is one hundred thousand dollars.

The small retailer or street peddler makes his money by adulterating the drug with powdered sugar or starch. The volume of drug traffic, according to *The Financial Times* article in 1985, is about twenty-five billion dollars a year. The circulation of such sums of money cannot go unnoticed by international financial circles. However, the finance ministers of the concerned countries are reticent about discussing this source of income which is not accounted for in their budgets. They represent two billion dollars for Colombia and one to one and a half billion for Bolivia and Peru. A portion of this income is invested in the United States or in Switzerland and another portion goes to the purchase of consumer goods by the big traffickers whose ranches, luxurious cars, and lavish residences are public knowledge. A fraction of that money is also invested in legitimate businesses in South America, thus allowing the big dealers to launder some drug money. More important, concludes *The Financial Times,* "All this money confers on certain individuals enough economic clout to wield their influence on the powers that be."

It is not South America alone that profits from drug money. Large North American banks plow important capital sums back into circulation, and it is symptomatic that in 1986 two of them, one in Boston and one in New York, received multi-million dollar fines for failing to report certain transactions with South America, as required by law. Not to be overlooked is the fact that North American banks have made mutli-billion dollar loans to South American governments, loans on which all they can presently collect is interest, and sometimes not even that. This interest adds up to billions of dollars, approximately the income South Americans derive from their cocaine trade. A brutal interruption of the cocaine traffic could worsen the foreign debt of the producer countries and lead them to bankrupcy.

However, one can hardly hold the South Americans solely responsible for the illegal consumption of cocaine by millions of North American citizens whose ever-growing fondness for the white powder has led five to six million of them to use it regularly at a rate of one hundred and thirty tons a year, according to the 1986 statistics released by the Drug Enforcement Administration. The most popular form of consumption is smoking cocaine base in the form of "crack," easily produced by combining cocaine hydrochloride with bicarbonate of soda. A crack epidemic is spreading throughout society, from floor sweepers to bank presidents and to all age groups from children to senior citizens.

John de Lorean, engineer, flamboyant businessman, and former vice-president of General Motors, decided in the early eighties to branch out on his own and invest in the construction of the car of the century. With the support of British financiers, he opened a factory in Northern Ireland. He ran into difficulties and was out of money before his first car left the assembly-line. One day, all America witnessed de Lorean on television toasting with champagne the purchase of a multi-million dollar cargo of cocaine. He had just concluded the exchange with undercover agents of the Drug Enforcement Agency, who promptly moved to arrest him. They had infiltrated the network used by de Lorean to make a cocaine deal in order to prop up his shaky business. He was trapped in a luxurious hotel room in Los Angeles where the transaction was filmed by hidden cameras.

His trial lasted for weeks and was widely publicized. Youthful Madame de Lorean, like a fashion model, wore a stunning new outfit everyday for the viewers to admire while she accompanied her husband to court. John de Lorean was defended by the best lawyers in the country. His line of defense was to prove entrapment by agents, former drug dealers, and have their testimony thrown out of court. Acquitted without ever having to appear on the witness stand, de Lorean "thanked God for having seen that justice was done."

In the minds of the California jurors, the dubious methods used by the agents violated the civil rights of the accused. This violation appeared more serious than the crime of dealing in drugs. Their decision, however, might have been influenced by the social acceptance of the drug in Los Angeles.

It appeared that the solemn warning voiced by Dr. Jeri at the Santa Monica Cocaine Symposium two years previously against the trivialization of cocaine recreational use had fallen on deaf ears. It did not stir up a pubic outcry in the United States sufficient to interdict the recreational use of this drug in any form. At the same time, thousands of articles and publications describing the dangers of cocaine use flooded the media. In 1984, Dr. Mark Gold, dedicated young psychiatrist in the

New York area, opened a free telephone line, "800 CO-
CAINE,"[10] to help cocaine addicts in distress. The hundreds
who called daily found a friendly ear and heard advice on how
to kick the habit, a most arduous task since it requires in many
cases an indefinite and often costly stay in a drug-free establishment. Cocaine addicts, often, have family and professional
responsibilities, which preclude prolonged periods of absence
from their work.

The efforts to disseminate information that would curb
the demand for cocaine or encourage addicts to seek rehabilitation have failed to check an epidemic which has reached levels
threatening to American society. Richard Smith, Chief Editor
of *Newsweek,* declared on June 16, 1986, that "America is
suffering from an epidemic as dangerous and widespread as the
medieval plague." Nowadays in the United States the social
acceptance of recreational drug use combined with the unequalled power of cocaine addiction all but cancel educational
efforts to decrease the American citizen's demand for the drug.

Efforts by the United States to reduce the sources of
production by strictly enforcing repressive policies were attempted in the summer of 1986. Light transport planes and
American agents were sent to Bolivia to assist the Bolivian
forces in destroying the cocaine laboratories which feed the
U.S. market. The operation failed, as the troops found nothing
except dismantled or abandoned laboratories. But it was sufficient to interrupt the traffic and the flow of cash into the
Bolivian treasury, which promptly requested a one hundred
million dollar indemnity from the United States to compensate
the losses incurred by the suspension of cocaine traffic.

Several weeks later, in the heart of the jungle, not far
from Tingo Maria, Peruvian planes blasted the clandestine
laboratories and the runways built by the traffickers that I had
seen from the air with the Cousteau team a few years earlier.
The plane intervened after the helicopters were shelled by
heavy gunfire from the ground. However, the limited incur-
sions of the Peruvian Army against the cocaine producers and
traffickers were short-lived and, like other similar interventions, did not decrease the flow of cocaine paste from the jungle
to the Colombian laboratories for long. Areas of cultivation
have steadily increased since 1986 in Peru and Bolivia, countries saddled by depressed economies, lacking political cohe-

sion, and, therefore, unable to stem the rising tide of coca production.

Concurrently, the drug lords of Medellin in Colombia are more powerful than ever and even have the upper hand in the war waged against them by the Colombian government. Their leader, 40-year-old Pablo Escobar, is, according to *Forbes Magazine,* the fourteenth-richest man in the world, with a fortune of $3 billion. He has assembled a grand operation with its own airfleet, security forces, export network, and chemists. The Medellin cartel (controlled by Escobar and his associates Carlos Lehder, now in prison, and Jorge Ochoa) which yearly grosses in excess of $5 billion, was responsible for the murder within four years of a minister of justice, an attorney general, more than fifty judges, and hundreds of policemen and soldiers. Nevertheless, the Colombian government has not sat back idly. For the first half of 1988 it reported the seizure of 14 tons of cocaine, the confiscation of 125,000 gallons of ether (used for the extraction of cocaine), the destruction of 684 labs, the dismantling of 39 airstrips, the arrest of 3500 people, and the sequestration of 30 planes. Yet this military campaign had little effect on the amount of cocaine reaching the consumers in the United States. The price of cocaine sold in American cities is at a record low: in 1980 a kilogram was worth $60,000 in Miami; in 1988 is sold for $14,000. The cocaine trade has become an international business, and the sources of production, limited until recently to Peru and Bolivia, are now surfacing in other South American countries. During a fact-finding visit to Brazil in 1987 I learned that the Epadu variety of the coca bush grows in the wild along the Amazon and could provide huge amounts of coca leaf. New routes of cocaine traffic towards Europe and the U.S. originate near the Brazilian megalopolis of São Paulo.

The solution to the problem, which is still growing, remains the same: the control of the sources of supply, as emphasized by the United States reform movement from Theodore Roosevelt to Stephen Porter, and as exemplified by the control of opium in China at the turn of the century. The cocaine-producing countries must plan a gradual eradication program of the coca bush plantations matched by the growing of basic food crops, fruit trees, and cocoa. We have seen that such an effort, which calls for considerable assistance staggered over many years, cannot be carried out by strictly bilateral agreements between North and South America. It will require the intervention of the United Nations, which had several decades ago formulated legislation for traffic interdiction, but which lacks the power and the international commitment to implement the legislation.

The United States cannot single-handedly win cocaine wars waged on several continents; it needs the support of all of its allies and of the country which has become its prime opponent after having helped it to win the Second World War. The European allies of the United States, who share its great democratic ideals, could help by rejecting the trivialization of drug use in their own countries instead of accepting it as inevitable and as a form of social progress. France, a privileged ally of the United States, and with its long tradition of defending human rights against oppression, can lead this cultural fight.

And, foremost, the United States must deal with the USSR, whose philosophy and culture are fundamentally opposed to drug use. The USSR has ratified all the international agreements designed to suppress illicit drug traffic and its recreational use. Until recently, the Soviets claimed that their progressive society was immune to illicit drug consumption, and, having no problem of their own, appeared indifferent to the major drug epidemics which swept through the western world. And it is true that illicit drug consumption, especially cocaine, even today, is very limited in the USSR when compared to what it is in the United States.

With *perestroika* ("openness"), *glassnost* ("restructuring"), and the unsealing of Soviet borders for greater international exchanges, the situation has changed and the people of the USSR are becoming more vulnerable to illicit drug addiction. On the southern borders of the USSR, Afghanistan, Iran, and Pakistan[10] are major producers of cannabis and opium, and many of the Soviet soldiers retreating from Afghanistan have been initiated in the consumption of these drugs.

On its western border, Poland may be considered as a model country for the development of an epidemic of drug dependence and especially of cannabis smoking and of heroin addiction. According to the Polish authorities I met in Warsaw late in 1988,[11] over a half million young Poles smoke home-grown cannabis and 40,000 are addicted to locally-produced heroin. Three main features are contributing to this epidemic of drug dependence: The country is in the throes of cultural and political ferment which favors the development of a libertarian counter-culture and of social nihilism. The government lacks popular support and is unable to enforce the repressive drug laws, which include the death penalty for the traffickers. Finally, the sources of supply, cannabis and the opium poppy, are grown domestically. Farms have not been collectivized and farmers own their land, so authorities have difficulty controlling the cultivation and processing of the opium poppy which is grown legally on over 8,000 acres for the production of morphine to supply the eastern bloc countries including the USSR.

I was shown some confiscated samples of the heroin brew prepared from diverted poppy straw and capsules which are boiled in water. Acetic acid, which transforms morphine into heroin, is added to this "soup," as it is called, and which after evaporation results in a mixture containing as much as 50% heroin. The tea-colored syrup is kept in small bottles capped with a syringe and used by the addicts for intravenous administration. In Warsaw I visited a detoxification center where eight addicts, very thin and pale, were being treated for withdrawal. Half of them were carriers of the AIDs virus. Public health officials are concerned about the transmission of the AIDS infection through sexual contact from the addicted to the non-addicted population.

Soviet leaders today must be concerned by the possible spread to their own restive youth of the consumption of cannabis and heroin which are produced and used in large amounts in adjoining lands. Heroin traffic represents today for the USSR a threat comparable to the cocaine menace for the United States: the producing countries are in their own backyard. Their concern must be a real one since the USSR signed a protocol with the U.S. in January of 1989 concerning the interdiction of the heroin traffic. This agreement could be the forerunner of global control of all illicit drugs including cocaine.

The war against cocaine will only be waged in earnest when the two big powers, having resolved some of the world's major confrontational issues, join forces in an international common front. It will then be possible to enforce the United Nations' laws which ban cocaine and heroin traffic but which have been defied and flaunted during the past twenty years.

International control of the sources of supplies of cocaine

associated with crop substitution will go a long way to implement the Single Convention of the United Nations of 1961, and also benefit the impoverished farmers and laborers of Peru, Bolivia, and Brazil. Once the sources of supply become unavailable for illicit traffic, the marketing organization of the Colombia Medellin Cartel will have to get out of business. This strategy to defeat the cocaine war lords might become a good illustration of the indirect approach described by Liddell Hart,[12] to beat a powerful enemy, and which has been a winning maneuver throughout history.

At the end of April 1989, the seizure in Miami of two tons of cocaine, the largest haul ever, on a Brazilian Varig airliner coming from Rio de Janeiro,[13] shows the urgency of controlling the production of this drug at its source. This seizure would indicate that cocaine is already being extracted in large amounts from the foliage of the Epadu tree which grows in the wild along the lower Amazon, and provides for a new, inexhaustible source of cocaine. If it is not controlled, an overflooding of the U.S. market, and a fast penetration of the Western European one, may rapidly occur.[14]

However a reversal in the policy of the Eastern bloc concerning the cocaine trade might have been heralded by Cuba in July of 1989. Ten years after it had condemned the trans–shipment of cocaine from Colombia to the U.S., the Castro régime condemned to death four of its prominent political and military figures, including a general, who were shot for abetting the cocaine trade. Should this dramatic move be considered as a new challenge to the West?

26

Experimental Administration of Cocaine to the Human and Nonhuman Primate

One year after Cousteau's team had completed its documentary, *Snowstorm in the Jungle,* I went back to Colombia and Peru. Some of the scientists I had met with Jean-Michel Cousteau had invited me back, and the State Department was funding and organizing my trip. Since 1908 the State Department has played a key role in the control of illicit drug traffic, which requires a close cooperation with the nations which produce the bulk of heroin or cocaine.[1] The policy of the State Department is based on international and bilateral treaties which ban the illicit traffic of controlled substances. As there are still no agreements for international control of the production of illicit drugs at their source, the State Department keeps reminding — diplomatically through its embassies — the producing countries of their obligations under existing treaties. Assistance is also offered to the producing countries in order to help them when they are ready to take measures aimed at curtailing illicit drug traffic and decreasing drug consumption. For this purpose one of the programs sponsored by the State Department through the United States Information Agency (U.S.I.A.) is to establish cultural exchanges of professional "expert" personnel experienced in the prevention of drug dependence.

I have been a frequent American participant ("AMPART," as we are called) in such programs and have found them very productive and most informative. Thanks to the efficiency of the embassy personnel and their excellently-planned scheduling, I have always been able to meet, within a few days, the principal government and nongovernment agencies in foreign countries which deal with illicit drug use and traffic and implement the various countermeasures which are taken. My contribution has been to present the medical and scientific aspects of drug dependence to the foreign audiences, and to discuss the different solutions which may be taken in the areas of prevention and rehabilitation. As a peripatetic scientist and as an AMPART I have visited many countries[2] in the Americas, Europe, the Middle East and the Far East. All of them are saddled with a very serious drug problem but none is so gravely affected as Bolivia, Colombia, and Peru because of the flourishing cocaine traffic and widespread coca paste consumption in those three nations.

Returning to Lima, Peru, in 1984, as an AMPART under the aegis of U.S.I.A., I called immediately on Raoul Jeri and we embraced warmly in South American style. With his unchanged quiet determination, Jeri was dedicated to the care of the growing number of cocaine victims he received in his hospital service at San Marcos University. He reminded me of Dr. Rieux, in Camus' *The Plague*,[3] who stoically attended the patients stricken by the fatal disease that decimated his home town.

"The situation is getting worse," he told me. "More and more coca paste is smoked, and at all ages! We have treated in my clinic old men over seventy-five and even addicted children who are four years old. Little boys no older than the one we saw smoking tobacco cigarettes in Juan Juy! Lately I have noticed in many coca smokers a whole new pathology: serious lung infections, meningitis, brain abscesses."

"Is the paste they smoke contaminated?"

"It is, with all kinds of bacteria and parasites."

As we reminisced about last years' expedition, I inquired about our Peruvian bodyguards.

Jeri shook his head sadly.

"The agents of the Peruvian Police Forces who accompanied us to Tingo Maria and Juan Juy were ambushed, one after another. Twelve were killed, one survived by playing dead, and another one was critically wounded."

"And young Captain Ramon who was with us through the whole trip?"

"He was shot several times and his brain was blown out, as if to make sure he wouldn't get away. The traffickers sent an explicit message to the Peruvian authorities: "No more filming in this area; the producers won't come out alive.' Cousteau was warned, of course."

"How about you, Raoul? You must be a target too, as the official doctor of the Peruvian police forces?"

"Well, I'm only a physician who treats the victims, and some of them are themselves traffickers."

During my stay in Lima, I gave a lecture to a group of health professionals in the concrete fortress where the American Cultural Services were housed. Dr. Hinojosa and Dr. Llosa, who were still performing cyngulotomies on *pastalaros,* attended my talk. I showed the film on the self-administration of cocaine by the rhesus monkey to illustrate the compulsive behavior of a primate with unlimited access to cocaine. After the film I spoke with Dr. Hinojosa.

"You've seen an experimental model which could be used to verify your theories. Would the primate continue to self-administer cocaine if it had been cyngulotomized?[4] Have you considered such an experiment?"

"No. You're the one who should be doing it because you have the equipment and all the funding. In Peru we could never find enough financial support for that kind of work. Moreover, we don't have the scientific experts needed to direct the studies. I'm willing to operate on all the monkeys you want, but it's up to you, the researchers, to do the rest."

For Hinojosa, the next move was up to American scientists. I didn't answer, but I had to admit he was right. Experimenting on a monkey which had been lobotomized could throw some light on the brain mechanisms which, when impaired by cocaine, induce a compulsive behavior and prevent the primate from performing functions essential for his survival. And yet this research had not been initiated in the specialized laboratories of the United States where the behavior of monkeys self–administering cocaine and other drugs of dependence had been systematically studied for nearly two decades, by outstanding scientists working with highly sophisticated equipment.

However, regulations concerning the use of animals for research had become most stringent in United States laboratories.[5] All studies, especially on primates, which could be associated with undue discomfort or pain were strictly scrutinized by committees created to meet the criticism of humane societies that opposed the indiscriminate use of animals in medical research. I doubt that Dr. Hinojosa would have understood all of the administrative difficulties and cultural obstacles that an American investigator would have encountered had he wanted to perform on monkeys the kind of surgical procedures carried out by Peruvian surgeons on man.

A year later I found that this restrictive policy governing nonhuman primate research was strictly observed at the Addiction Research Center of the National Institute on Drug Abuse in Baltimore.[6] As a visiting scientist, I studied the effects of antidotes to cocaine in the squirrel monkey. The amount of drug administered to the animal had been carefully calculated so as to be far below the dose which could produce toxic effects such as convulsions or cardiac failure. The selected dose was administered to the animal only every three weeks. I was also informed that the squirrel monkeys imported from South America were quite valuable, worth over $1,000 each. Nevertheless, the relatively small dose of cocaine administered to the monkey induced marked increases in blood pressure and heart rate as well as brief irregularities of the heart which were indicative of transient suffering in the cardiac muscle.[7] These acute changes could be neutralized by the same antidotes which we had used to protect rats against the damaging lethal effects of cocaine.[8]

At the same time, other medical scientists at the Addiction Research Center were studying the effects of cocaine administered to man. Paid volunteers, who were also confirmed cocaine addicts, were injected with doses of cocaine sufficient to produce increased heart rate and blood pressure, and to induce euphoria and tolerance. The drug was given either in successive small doses or in larger doses over a longer period of time in order to prevent toxic accumulation.

Such experiments duplicated to a great extent those performed at the University of Chicago in the late seventies by a group of American scientists led by Dr. Charles Schuster and Marion Fischman.[9] After observing that human volunteers, all cocaine addicts, when given the opportunity, not only inject themselves with cocaine rather than with salt water but also tend to increase the dose rapidly, these researchers concluded that "Human experiments confirm the reinforcement action of cocaine leading to a behavior of frequent consumption. Similar studies conducted on monkeys are less valuable than those performed on humans." Such studies on man, entirely supported with public funds amounting to several million dollars, have continued to this day.[10] These experiments, performed under controlled laboratory conditions, provide little information which was not already known from the careful clinical observations reported by Maier and Lewin at the turn of the century.

Such human studies made me feel quite uncomfortable, especially after I learned from one of the researchers at the Addiction Research Center that several of the subjects who were administered a slow continuous infusion of cocaine had displayed measurable symptoms of paranoia. I voiced my objections to these human studies to the Director of the Center,[11] who disagreed with me, as did the director of the National Institute on Drug Abuse.[12] I had a chance to formulate my objections to the Advisory Board of the National Institute on Drug Abuse,[13] which also disagreed with my position. They all referred to the recommendations of a 1987 ad hoc committee of investigators on drug dependence,[14] which assembled a most competent group of thirty-two leading pharmacologists and psychiatrists. The committee recommended the continuation of experimental studies in which cocaine is administered to cocaine addicts under controlled conditions. It was argued that such studies would yield "sorely needed information relevant to treatment of cocaine addicts." One of the members of the committee had previously expressed the following opinion: "Some preliminary research questions may be tested by giving opiates, stimulant drugs, to non-drug users for a long enough period of time to produce a sufficient state of dependence."[15]

I was also informed that all of the studies funded by NIDA to study the effects of cocaine on man underwent a stringent critical peer review including protection of human subjects. The project also had to be approved at the researcher's institution by an institutional review board, which included other researchers as well as physicians and laymen who made sure that human subjects would not be exposed to risks greater than the benefits that were expected to be derived from carrying out the research project. Finally, all human research utilizing new applications for old drugs were approved by the Food and Drug Administration.

In spite of this massive approval schedule for the continued funding of studies of cocaine administration to man, I was
firmly opposed to this practice. A thorough review of the recent
medical literature and experimental observations made in my
laboratory confirmed my misgivings. In the American literature alone I found ten reports of 140 cocaine-related deaths
following recreational use of the drug between 1975 and 1985.
Since 1986, additional reports have related recreational use of
cocaine to cerebral vessel damage.[16]

No such accident has ever been reported in studies of
human cocaine addicts who are carefully screened from a large
pool of applicants for their good physical and mental health
and given thorough physical and psychiatric examinations. But
still, subtle microscopic damage to blood vessels of the brain
and heart might be produced by even small amounts of cocaine—damage which may not be detectable by routine
methods of monitoring such as electrocardiogram and mood
scale measurements currently used on subjects to whom cocaine is administered.

One paper, *Cocaine and the Heart,* published in 1987,[17]
described the presence of microscopic rupture of strands of
heart muscles in 93% of apparently normal hearts removed
from subjects whose deaths were cocaine-related. Similar lesions, called "contraction band necroses," were observed in
patients who had succumbed after brief periods of decreased
blood and oxygen supply to the heart, often caused by an
excessive amount of substances like adrenalin which make the
blood vessels constrict.

In my own laboratory we had observed that cardiac lesions produced by large doses of cocaine were related to the
release in the bloodstream of substances such as adrenaline and
angiotensin which produce a narrowing of blood vessels and
hypertension.[18] Our studies led us to discover medications that
protect the animal against lethal doses of cocaine by preventing
massive discharge of these pressor agents into the circulation.
We had concluded that over the long run damage could be
caused to the small blood vessels of the heart and brain by the
repetitive biochemical and pressure changes induced by cocaine. Experimental evidence from the older literature, which
was already mentioned, and more recent studies, indicated
that cocaine could also have a damaging effect on the liver,[19]
kidney, and the immune system, mainly as a result of the

massive release of adrenalin–like substances produced by the drug in vessels and tissues.

I could not see the benefits resulting from human experiments with cocaine that would offset their potential danger. Studies should first be performed on animals administered small doses of cocaine repetitively, similar to the manner in which cocaine is being given to the human "volunteers." The animals, unlike humans, could be euthanized and microscopic examination of brain, heart, kidney, and liver specimens performed using new staining techniques. Special studies should be directed at identifying "myocardial band necrosis"[20] and vascular lesions of heart.

The subjects actually selected for the human studies are paid cocaine addicts, a point which raises legal as well as ethical problems. Under the law a physician is allowed to administer controlled substances for the purpose of treating an ailment; in the case of cocaine, it is legally used only to induce local surface anesthesia. Cocaine administration to cocaine addicts for experimental purposes might be an infringement of the Harrison Act[21] (see Chapter 10). The broad interpretation of this Act, sustained twice by the Supreme Court (1919, 1926), forbids a physician to prescribe for other than medicinal purposes any of the drugs falling under the jurisdiction of the Act (opiates and cocaine). The Supreme Court ruling specifically forbids a physician to prescribe an addictive drug to an addict, thus maintaining his addiction.[22]

In the present situation, the purpose of cocaine administration to an addict as performed by NIDA scientists is to find some scientific clues which might lead to a cure. However, it is questionable that such an empirical open–ended approach will ever reach such a lofty goal. It has been pursued for more than a decade and has brought to the fore very little new knowledge, while perpetuating the addiction of the experimental subjects. It is my opinion that this approach, which carries some risk to the subject, lacks a conceptual as well as a physiological basis, discussed in the following chapter.

In addition to the legal issue involved for the physician, there is an ethical one: to justify giving cocaine to a cocaine addict. Cocaine administration will further reinforce the addictive behavior which the physician would like to help the addict give up.

Finally, these human studies might be conflicting with the

following recommendations from the Helsinki Declaration on Human Rights concerning "Non-Therapeutic Clinical Research.[23]

> The subject of clinical research should be in such a mental physical and legal state as to be able to exercise fully his power of choice.
> The investigator must respect the right of each individual to safeguard his personal integrity especially if the subject is in a dependent relationship to the investigator.

These recommendations raise the two following questions: Is an addict, dependent on cocaine and paid to inject his drug of dependence, in a position to "exercise fully his power of choice"? Is an addict, dependent on cocaine and given cocaine by the investigator, in a dependent relationship to the investigator?

I therefore remained convinced that, all things considered, the experimental administration of cocaine to cocaine addicts should not be pursued. Instead, research should be directed towards studies on animal preparations in order to investigate the effects of cocaine on some of the basic mechanisms of heart and brain which are impaired by the drug. These mechanisms can only be pinpointed by acute and chronic studies on rats and mice, using, at times toxic doses of cocaine which therefore may not be used in human experimentation.

New medications may then be tested on these same animal models to neutralize or mitigate the toxic effects of cocaine and counteract the impairment induced by the drug on vital functions. The medications proven effective and safe experimentally may then be used to wean the cocaine addict from the drug and enable the addict to tolerate withdrawal symptoms better.

This traditional therapeutic approach is aimed at speeding the recovery of the addict and helping him to achieve a drug free life instead of perpetuating his addiction. This addiction may be defined today as a self-inflicted impairment of brain function.

27

Cocaine Addiction, A Self–Inflicted Impairment of Brain Neurotransmission

It is clear that man has a limited power to control the intake of cocaine once he has started using the drug. Compulsive drug–consuming behavior, which is also displayed by other mammals, may be attributed to the inherent property of cocaine to stimulate in a most rapid and potent fashion brain mechanisms which induce feelings of pleasure and reward. These brain mechanisms, identified in man by the great American neurologist Robert Heath,[1] are centered in the limbic system of the old primitive brain which controls drives and emotions and favors the dominant activities of nutrition and reproduction essential for survival of the individual and the species. The Old Brain is entirely surrounded by the New Brain, or neocortex, which is the center of intelligence, symbolic expression, and self–consciousness. Old and New Brain are closely knit to one another, and their respective activities are highly integrated and complement each other at every moment.

We often assume that "the power of reason" expressed through the neocortex is dominant and will keep in check the strong impulses of the Old Brain, a mere assumption, as the French scientist and philosopher Blaise Pascal tells us in his famous saying of 300 years ago: "The heart has its own reasons that Reason does not know."[2] Pascal did not realize at the time, like many of us today, that the heart he was referring to was "located" in the limbic part of the brain, but he was able to formulate the basic duality of the human brain.

The extraordinary miracle of the human brain rests in its capacity to express itself in a coherent, reasonable fashion by integrating and balancing the activities of its "emotional" old part and its "rational" new part. To this effect every thousandth of a second the brain prioritizes and marshals myriads of signals according to modalities that adjust to the conditions of the environment and to its own memory banks. Cocaine seems to destabilize these two parts of the brain by amplifying the signals arising from the Old Brain and distorting those emanating from the New Brain.[3] All of these signals are chemically transmitted through minute quantities of substances called neurotransmitters which are secreted by billions of nerve cells or "neurons." Neurotransmitters will regulate the transmission of nerve impulses racing through the cerebral network, across a hundred billion relays or "synapses." Cocaine perturbs and may even damage biochemical regulations which allow the normal turnover of the key neurotransmitters, norepinephrine and dopamine, to take place in the areas of the Old Brain which have been associated with pleasure–reward.[4] These substances are continuously secreted in the form of granules by nerve switches or synapses to ensure the passage of information from one cell to another. The neurotransmitter granules are also recaptured by the cellular membrane that has secreted them. Secretion and reuptake of chemical messages occur in billions of synapses, billions of times per fraction of a second. Cocaine stimulates the production of noradrenaline and dopamine at the synaptic membrane, while preventing their recapture, and so these key neurotransmitters accumulate, reaching concentrations that first impair, and may even, in the long run, damage the function of the limbic brain.

We observed in our laboratory[5] that cocaine induces cardiac lesions resulting from the damage to the heart cells by an excess of these neurotransmitter substances. We used an antidote which neutralizes the effects of these substances and were able to preserve the integrity of the heart cells. Similar events can be expected to take place in brain cells, which are known to produce excessive amounts of norepinephrine and dopamine under the influence of cocaine. We were able to demonstrate that the toxicity of cocaine is, to a great extent, indirect. The experiments showed that cocaine itself, although present, is not what causes the toxicity. Rather, toxicity is due to the marked increase in production of neurotransmitter substances that cocaine induces.

The brain is also continuously producing the same neurotransmitters in order to maintain its proper functioning. Under the influence of cocaine the production of these neurotransmitters increases and an acute, most pleasant, state of hyperexcitability occurs; when the administration of the drug is repeated, addiction will develop, the brain being forced to function at a high level of rewarding activity, which may be maintained only by more cocaine. Such a mechanism could explain the compulsive aspect of cocaine addiction.

My colleague Lucien Cote, a professor of neurology at Columbia University, has documented the progressive decrease in dopamine–containing nerve cells which occurs during a lifetime, from a maximal number during adolescence to half as many at age sixty.[6] This fact might account for the ebullience, energy, and hyperactivity of youth, and also for their greater vulnerability to cocaine which will trigger the many doapminergic cells that are all set to move into high gear.

Cocaine interferes with transmission through the brain somewhat as extraneous noises distort messages on the airwaves. In French these noises are called "parasites." One might wonder whether it would be possible to rid the brain of its chemical parasites by neutralizing them with another chemical substance. Such a "brain penicillin" could restore the balance impaired by the drug and chemically condition the free play of the mental faculties, thus directing the individual toward rational behavior. This possibility was suggested in 1979 by Arthur Koestler[7] who saw in it the only way to preserve the survival of Homo sapiens, eternal victim of the destructive instincts of his old brain. In his book *Janus* Koestler suggested that new chemical substances created by psycho–pharmacologists ought to be able to repress the aggressive tendencies of an individual and allow his rational mind to express itself freely. We have seen that it is possible to neutralize the acute effects of cocaine by administering specific chemicals. But this treatment is only temporary and does not eliminate the memory of the pleasant intoxicating experience which seems imprinted on the brain as a very compelling memory.

Biochemical restoration of normal brain function may not be readily achieved because it is the result of innumerable chemically interdependent regulations which must take place in an internal environment with a stable chemical composition. As Claude Bernard[8] wrote in his *Introduction to Experimental Medicine* in 1874, "The constancy of the internal environment is the condition for a free life." The American physiologist Walter Cannon[9] elevated this axiom into a general law by coining a new word, "homeostasis," to describe the natural equilibrium of the regulations essential to survival.

The brain is, of all the organs of the human body, the one where the "homeostasis" principle applies most perfectly. The stability of the chemical composition of its internal environment, a fluid in which billions of neurons are immersed, is the very condition of their coherent activity. But cocaine alters the recycling of substances secreted by brain cells in order to transmit a free flow of coherent messages. This wondrous, self-regulating performance of the brain, resting on internal recycling, is first altered, then damaged, by cocaine.

Finally, if it were possible to use drug treatment to permanently restore the balance of a brain perturbed by cocaine, it would also seem possible to chemically condition human behavior, as the Peruvian psychiatrist tries to do with "astronaut vitamins."

Nature has so engineered the brain that such a chemical manipulation appears doomed to failure. A balanced expression of the intellectual and emotional functions of the brain may only occur within a cerebral environment with a composition delicately regulated by the cyclical renewal of its neurotransmitters. The only way to treat cocaine addiction is therefore to cleanse the brain and retrain it to function without the drug. Nothing but complete abstinence can restore the well-balanced internal milieu needed for continuous normal brain performance.

Abstinence is made possible by the extraordinary resiliency of the brain and its spontaneous tendency to recover its balance when the acute effect of the drug wears off. The periodic return, after drug intoxication, to a normal state frequently gives the addict, and those close to him, the impression that he can stop using the drug when and if he really wants to. But the reprieve is short and the withdrawal symptoms appear, enticing the addict to return to his poison so that the brain can continue to operate in the new neuro-chemical conditions caused by the drug. Furthermore, the pleasant experience associated with the consumption of cocaine has imprinted a most dominant memory on the brain, so dominant that it will lead a former addict, who has been abstinent for years, to consume the drug again, if it is made available to him.

The presence of this affective memory associated with cocaine use explains why a rehabilitated addict may never be considered "cured," since he will not be able to consume this drug again without reverting to his addiction. The same may be said about other addictive drugs such as opiates, and even alcohol or tobacco. All individual experiences are imprinted on the brain in the form of memories which, when considered in their entirety, determine the personality of each individual and to a great extent his behavior. Certain memories evoke pleasant feelings which may even harken back to many years past. One of the best illustrations of such fond memories is that recalled by the French writer Marcel Proust[10] in his book *Remembrance of Things Past*. While dipping a little bun in warm tea sweetened with sugar and milk, the aging author is reminded of the delightful feelings of sweetness and warmth which he experienced as a child when a loving aunt provided him with the same little treat in the late afternoon. Cocaine marks the brain with a biochemically imprinted memory called an "engram" that may not be erased.

Some intellectuals have claimed that the freedom of the cocaine addict to consume his drug of choice should be respected. But is it not a delusion to speak of the freedom of the addict who has, in fact, become the slave of a substance that disrupts the normal chemistry of his brain which has become unable to exert its rational function? Because of its specific impairing properties on brain mechanisms, cocaine curtails the exercise of free will. Today the scientist is in a position to measure the fallacy of John Stuart Mill's general statement: "Over himself, over his own body and mind, the individual is sovereign"[11] when it applies to cocaine consumption. The exercise of freedom requires a relationship of authenticity between the brain and the surrounding environment, as stated in 1858 by the French poet, Baudelaire,[12] long before the scientist: "It is forbidden to man, under threat of degradation and spiritual death, to disrupt the equilibrium which prevails between his mental faculties and the environment in which they express themselves, in other words, tamper with one's own destiny and place it under another kind of fate." And here Baudelaire was referring to the disrupting effect of hashish on the mind which he had experienced but refused to pursue.

We may recall that the frailty of the balance of brain regulations was described by the French psychiatrist, Joseph

Moreau,[13] a hundred and fifty years ago: "What brain alterations, what reordering of brain molecules can be linked to the mistaken notions, the false beliefs which all of us harbor, whether dunce or scholars?"

Cocaine distorts the natural interplay of basic brain regulations which depend on a normal recycling of chemical substances produced by our body to maintain a coherent brain function. Affected by the drug, these natural substances will reach a toxic level which prevents the expression of the rational mind. By its crippling effects on the delicate and fine balance of brain regulations, cocaine will "elicit the mistaken beliefs we all harbor."

By inducing in the brain a new biochemical regimen and "imprinting" a dominating memory which supersedes all others, cocaine establishes patterns of behavior solely oriented towards unending self–gratification. In some cases such brain alterations appear to be irreversible. As a result man may be transformed into a drug–seeking robot.

The presence in a society of many individuals hopelessly addicted to cocaine and unable to exert their free will result in damaging social effects, as documented by a study of history and also by the science of epidemiology.

28

The Epidemic Spread of Cocaine Addiction and its Containment

The compulsive drug-seeking behavior produced by cocaine and explained by the changes in brain chemistry induced by the drug is also illustrated by the science of "epidemiology," or the study of epidemics. Indeed, the "recreational" use of cocaine, like that of other addictive drugs, spreads in an epidemic fashion, as the Swedish sociologist Nils Bejerot clearly documented in his classical treatise *Addiction and Society.*[1]

Bejerot was the first to study and describe the "epidemic type of drug dependence" which has affected mostly adolescents and young adults of industrialized societies since the end of World War II. This type of addiction is different from the "professional type" and the "therapeutic type." The professional type affects health professionals and physicians in particular who have an easy access to addictive drugs. Incidence of addiction among physicians is, according to Bejerot, 30 to 50 times that of the general population. The "therapeutic type" of addiction affects patients who have become addicted through medication with dependence–producing drugs, and it prevailed widely in the United States at the turn of the century.

The epidemic type of youthful drug addiction was studied by Bejerot in Sweden, his home country, which in the sixties and seventies was swept by an epidemic of amphetamine abuse that affected the younger section of the population aged 15 to 25. The most essential feature of this epidemic type of addiction, writes Bejerot, is its "psychosocial contagion."

> The addict spreads the addictive behavior (injection of heroin or amphetamine, snorting cocaine or smoking crack) and the use of drugs to friends and sexual partners. Closeness of contact

with confirmed addicts constitutes the decisive factor in initiating addiction and is far more important than individual proneness to norm–breaking behavior. Tendency to spread addictive behavior is greatest at the beginning of an addiction career, particularly during the first year, which is called the "honeymoon of addiction."

In the Swedish epidemic, amphetamine, a major psychostimulant, was mostly intravenously injected. This mode of administration induces an intense rush and other symptoms like those of injected cocaine, as well as rapid, compelling, drug–seeking behavior. The amphetamine class of compounds are synthetic substances which were developed before World War II and introduced into therapy as stimulating medications, with many obvious widespread applications. They possess properties similar to those of cocaine: increasing wakefulness and alertness and elevating mood and self confidence, while depressing the appetite. Like cocaine they are dependence–producing drugs and induce marked tolerance; the withdrawal symptoms are manifested by depression and fatigue which occur when the consumer is deprived of the drug. The addictive power of amphetamine and its ability to induce an epidemic of addiction similar to that of cocaine is meticulously documented by the studies of Bejerot carried out over twenty–five years in Stockholm and other large Swedish cities. "This drug epidemic," writes the Swedish epidemiologist,

> provides an experimental model for studies of incidence of illicit drug abuse in function of the availability of the drug. Our studies demonstrate that a permissive drug policy leads to rapid spread of drug abuse: when there are plenty of drugs and the risks are small even addicts who have been off drugs for many years may relapse. A restrictive drug policy may not only check the spread of addiction, but even bring about a considerable reduction in the rate of current consumption in the addict population.

These conclusions were based on systematic surveys made by Bejerot and his colleagues among all persons arrested for criminal offenses in Stockholm between 1965 and 1987, 250,000 in all. Amphetamine users were recognized among all the arrestees by the needle marks that they presented on their arms. The progression or regression of the epidemic was gauged in calculating the percentage of addicts (marked with needle scars) among the population arrested for any kind of criminal or civil offense.

Until 1945 there were only a dozen or so drug addicts using amphetamine and heroin among bohemian circles of Stockholm. The intravenous mode of administration was then propagated by prostitutes and reached all of the marginal fringes of society. From then on the epidemic spread out steadily, doubling every thirty months until the estimated number of addicts reached 4,000 in 1965, with a parallel increase in criminality. Until that time the Swedish policy of controlling drug addiction was based on law enforcement, which was singled out by a group of social reformers as the very cause of the epidemic. A well-orchestrated media campaign called for a medical rather than a criminal approach to addiction, and in 1965 the Swedish Board of Health sanctioned an experiment of medical prescription of amphetamines (or of heroin) to addicts for self-administration. The percentage of amphetamine addicts among arrestees increased from 20 to 40 percent between 1965 and 1968. At that time the medical experiment of providing drugs to addicts was interrupted and a restrictive policy reinstated. The number of addicts dropped sharply, especially after an amphetamine distribution network was dismantled in 1972. By then the epidemic had spread to all Swedish large cities and to Norway and Denmark. "However," adds Bejerot, "most Swedish drug offenders could usually leave the police precinct after interrogation and were generally punished by fines, suspended sentences or psychiatric treatment. Thus the basic conditions for the spread of the epidemic remained and the epidemic began to increase again, with opiates compounding the amphetamine epidemic." Furthermore, many of the thousands of amphetamine and morphine addicts initiated during the experimental period of medical prescription were still to be counted in the addicted population some ten years later. As a result of the twin influence of greater availability and a residual pool of hard-core addicts from the 1965-68 epidemic, a new surge in addiction flared up after 1972, culminating in 1976 when 60 percent of all arrestees were diagnosed with needle marks. Restrictive drug laws were strengthened in 1977, and the percentage of needle addicts was brought down to 40 percent of all law-breakers in Stockholm. They numbered between 12,000 and 14,000, a figure which has remained stable, until 1988 at least, and which seems to be acceptable to Swedish authorities and to public opinion.

Bejerot contrasts the handling of the Swedish epidemic of

amphetamine abuse to the way the Japanese coped with a similar epidemic in the fifties: while the Swedes were able to stabilize the epidemic only at a relatively high level, the Japanese suppressed it nearly entirely.[2] The Japanese soldiers and especially their kamikaze pilots consumed large amounts of amphetamine during the Second World War. After the war these central stimulants were sold over the counter in Japan. Production of the drug increased; so did its consumption, and, as a result, numerous cases of addiction were reported. The amphetamines were then classified as dangerous drugs to be only prescribed by physicians. But thousands had already been addicted, and a widespread illegal fabrication and traffic of the drug occurred. At the height of the epidemic, in 1954, it was estimated that 2 million Japanese out of a population of 100 million consumed amphetamine tablets, and that 500,000 self-injected the drug intravenously, a situation far more serious than in Sweden at any time.

Under strong government leadership, Japanese public opinion was mobilized by the media to fight amphetamine addiction and accept the drastic measures required to stop the epidemic. Supply was curtailed by strictly controlling availability of amphetamines as well as the chemicals used for their fabrication. Conviction for illicit manufacture carried a ten-year jail sentence. Severe penalties were meted out to decrease the demand: three to six months in jail for use or possession, two to four years for sale, and five to ten years for traffic. In 1954, the first year of the antidrug campaign, 55,600 persons were arrested for drug related offenses. In 1956 there were 271 arrests, and the epidemic was checked. Convicted addicts were not referred to out-patient treatment centers but confined in jails or in specialized detention centers.

Later, in the 1960's, Japan faced (as did western nations) an epidemic of heroin addiction, involving at its peak an estimated 50,000 people. The Narcotics Control Law was amended with a two-pronged approach: To decrease the supply of heroin, life imprisonment for traffickers and seizure of their assets were instituted; to decrease demand, a system of compulsory hospitalization and rehabilitation of users was established. Within four years, the number of arrests for heroin use was cut from a high of 2,200 to less than 100 and has since remained at that low level.

Dr. Norbus Motohashi, head of Japan's Narcotics Division of the Ministry of Health, said in 1973, "To become a narcotic addict is an anti-social act and the foundation of countermeasures against addiction is to treat and rehabilitate addicts."[3]

In taking such drastic measures to stamp out drug addiction, the Japanese were aware of the damaging effects wrought by the widespread opiate consumption on the social fabric and national integrity of China in the 19th century. In the early part of the 19th century, British mercantilism imported opium from India to China to pay for tea and silk. In 1830, the Chinese leadership became alarmed and refused to allow the trade to continue. This was taken by the British as a cause for war, and two Opium Wars ensued in which the Chinese were defeated. The treaty of Tianjin in 1858 imposed on China an open-door trade policy including opium. A massive epidemic of opium use ensued among the Chinese people: imported opium rose from 325 tons in 1820 to 6,200 tons in 1873. A period of overwhelming opium addiction resulted which drained the faltering Chinese economy, and the Chinese, who could not buy all the drug from abroad, had to remove the ban on local cultivation. At the end of the 19th century, out of a population of 300 million Chinese, 90 million were addicted to opium; the old Chinese empire was threatened by fragmentation and the foreign powers were poised, ready to divide it into economic zones of influence. The dismantling did not occur. During the first part of the 20th century a national revival stressing the basic Chinese values prevailed in the country and restored China, 50 years later, to the rank of a world power. It was a period of revolution and civil strife pitting traditionalists against reformers, nationalists against communists. But in spite of their conflicting political allegiances, all of the Chinese were united in their determination to stamp out opium addiction from their country. In this endeavor they received the support of the United States and of the European powers.[4]

In 1906, a few years before the demise of the Manchu imperial dynasty, the Chinese government concluded the ten-year agreement with India that specified that China should cease domestic cultivation of poppies and forbid the consumption of opium on the understanding that the export of Indian opium to China should be reduced in equal proportion and cease altogether within a decade.

This bilateral agreement, which reversed a longstanding

British policy in India, was given added impetus by the Shanghai International Opium Conference held in 1911 at the suggestion of Theodore Roosevelt. Britain and France were among the thirteen world powers represented at the conference, which marks the beginning of an international policy aimed at restricting the use of opium to medical and scientific purposes only.

The convergent national and international measures directed against the opium trade were quite effective in curtailing opiate addiction among the Chinese people. At the 1917 meeting of the Opium Advisory Committee, the British representative Sir John Jordan could declare: "China has almost freed itself from the curse of the opium poppy."[5]

The Japanese were keenly aware of the damaging effects of opiates on the social fabric and political stability of China. In the 1930's, after conquering Manchuria from China, they reintroduced the cultivation of poppy to the Chinese mainland. Conversely, in 1942 when the Japanese wrested Indonesia from its Dutch colonial rulers, they destroyed the plantations of coca bush planted to manufacture cocaine for medical use abroad. In this case, they wanted to protect their soldiers against an addictive substance. Such examples indicate that addictive drugs may be used effectively as auxiliary weapons to wage war, only to weaken one's prospective enemy.

The total eradication of the use of opium from China only occurred at the end of the civil war in 1949, when Mao Tse-Tung assumed power over a unified country. The entire territory, including the former international concessions and the southern provinces, was made drug-free within a few years. However, in 1961 cultivation of opium resumed in Yunnan province, along the borders of the Golden Triangle, as reported by Professor Schipper. In one of the twists of history, China was now exporting opium to the western world. According to Heikal, a confidant of Nasser, Chou en Lai, the Chinese Premier, declared during a visit to the Egyptian leader in 1972: "The Chinese have not forgotten the Opium Wars, and are now poised to take advantage of the addictions which are plaguing the western world."[6]

Following their defeat in 1947, the Chinese nationalists retreated to Formosa (Taiwan) where the cultivation of the poppy had been banned since 1945, after the surrender of Japan. The Chinese in Taiwan, like those on the mainland, share the same contempt for opium and other addictive drugs. The Chinese were able to solve their problem of massive opium addiction by decreasing the demand for the drug and concurrently cutting off the supply. The demand for opium was curtailed when a national consensus against the drug finally surfaced at the turn of the century. This national consensus was independent from political allegiances. It was an ethical Chinese commitment which started under the imperial dynasty and continued under the Republic, the Kuomintang, and the Communists. Opium addiction has been eliminated in mainland China and Taiwan as well as Singapore. It still prevails only in Hong Kong, a British Crown Colony.

In stark contrast with Japan and China, Australia has failed to control an epidemic of illicit drug consumption which has swept this young and dynamic country since the early seventies. It all started with marijuana smoking. The locally grown cannabis plant provided large amounts of the drug and was supplemented by the stronger Buddha "sticks" and hashish blocks imported from Malaysia and Thailand. In 1977 the Senate Committee on Social Welfare concluded, on the basis of available surveys, that as many as 400,000 Australians, or about 3% of the total population, smoked cannabis at least once a month and that use of the drug was three to five times higher among adolescents and young adults.[7]

The trivialization of recreational marijuana smoking rapidly became as widely spread as it is in the United States and was followed by an epidemic of intravenous heroin use. In Sydney more than 20,000 addicts were identified in 1984,[8] when I first visited Australia. I had been invited by a group of concerned parents, on what had become for me a sort of world wide crusade against addictive drugs. A year later the prime minister of Australia, Robert Hawke, made a nationwide televised dramatic plea to warn the Australian people against using addictive drugs. In the course of his talk he informed his audience that his daughter was addicted to heroin and had given birth to an addicted baby. The same year a young Australian man was condemned to death and hanged in Malaysia for heroin traffic. These dramatic examples have done little to contain the epidemics of cannabis and opiate use in Australia. Cannabis consumption is for all practical purposes decriminalized, and a vocal movement supported by journalists and academics is pushing for its legalization as well as that of other addictive drugs. The heroin epidemic continues unabated in spite of increased seizures of the drug and free methadone programs. In 1988 death by opiate overdose in Sydney reached the figure of 126, an all-time high.

Australia has been spared until now from a cocaine epidemic, most probably because of its geographical location, separated as it is from the producing countries by the Pacific Ocean. Commercial exchanges are few and transportation links are also limited between Australia and South America.

By contrast, Spain, which has multiple direct ocean and air links with South America, has a major problem of cocaine usage, including that of crack in the past five years. In 1988, one ton of cocaine was seized in Barcelona, and one in San Sabastian. Addiction to this drug has compounded the current epidemic of heroin and of marijuana usage, the latter fanned by its decriminalization.[9]

It is now clear that the law enforcement model of controlling the epidemic type of drug addiction to heroin and to psychostimulants is most effective and requires a goal close to "zero tolerance" of drug addiction. This goal may be reached by a disciplined and structured society. The "medical" model which consists in providing the addict with his drug of choice, in order to eliminate criminality, has merely aggravated the problem in Sweden as well as in England where it was first adopted.

The British were the first, in 1925, to adopt a medical model allowing physicians to prescribe heroin to heroin addicts. This "British system" worked satisfactorily as long as addicts were few in number and all registered: 400 a year between 1930 and 1960. It became unmanageable after 1960, when heroin had to be dispensed to more than 1,000 users of the drug. Each addict had to be provided with daily doses of heroin, as well as the equipment required for the injection of the drug four to six times a day. Because of this logistical problem and because of the potential for diversion of the drug to nonregistered addicts, heroin began to be progressively replaced by methadone maintenance. (Methadone, a long-lasting opiate, needs to be absorbed only once a day, and by mouth.) But the number of registered British addicts had grown to 2,800 by 1980, double the total seeking treatment seven years earlier.[10] In 1985 there were an estimated 80,000 heroin addicts in Britain, most of whom were not in drug-treatment programs. Despite this failure of the British system, it is still advocated by some in the United States.

But the successful control of epidemics of drug addiction was also achieved by western nations. We have seen that widespread addiction to cocaine and opiates as a result of free availability of medications containing these drugs prevailed in the United States in the first part of the century. A 1915 health survey reported that there were 250,000 habitual users of cocaine or opiates in the nation with its population of 100 million. An aroused public opinion and the enlightened leadership of the progressives resulted in interdiction measures following the implementation of the Harrison Act to control the epidemic (see Chapter 10).

It should not be forgotten that during the period 1923 to 1939 the number of addicts was reduced to approximately 50,000, which represents an 80% drop, and in reference to the population of the country a 90% decrease.[11] This dramatic reduction was achieved by a restrictive control policy, with minimal education or medical intervention. A social refusal of illicit recreational drug use prevailed in the country. A similar popular consensus supported the restrictive policies which rolled back cocaine epidemics in Germany, France, and Switzerland after the First World War.

In the course of history, at times the use of cannabis, cocaine, or opiates has reached the "epidemic stage" which is characterized by widespread social acceptance and consumption. Hashish was widely and legally consumed in the Moslem world between the 12th and 16th centuries, as described by Fritz Rosenthal in his scholarly treatise, *The Herb Hashish versus Moslem Medieval Society.*[12] As a result, according to the contemporary historian Al Magrizy, a general debasement of a large segment of the population was apparent. When restrictive measures were finally applied the habit of hashish–taking had become so ingrained in the people that it would not be altogether eliminated. We have seen[13] that the consumption of opium also assumed an endemic form in China at the end of the 19th century, and while consumption of opiates was later eliminated from China, it continued, along with cultivation of the poppy, in adjoining Burma, Laos, and Thailand, the Golden Triangle countries which still are the major illegal producers and exporters of raw opium for the manufacture of heroin.[14] The chewing of coca leaves is still endemic in the

Peruvian and Bolivian Andes, where this custom is socially accepted and widely practiced. The anthropologist William Carter reports that ninety to ninety-five percent of *coqueiros* consume large amounts of coca leaves daily, as much as a man can chew in a day, and would revolt if they were deprived of their drug.[15] Even consumed in this self-limiting manner, by masticating the leaf, cocaine is addictive. As a result of this habit, the farmers and miners of the Andes are able to work under adverse conditions with limited food intake. Their social status has not changed in centuries. Their general health and life expectancy are poor. No one could have predicted that by an ironic twist of history the presence of this coca-chewing population and their need for consuming the apparently harmless coca leaf would be at the origin of the devastating cocaine epidemic of coca paste smoking which, after starting in Peruvian cities, has swept the Americas in the past ten years.

The consumption of alcohol, one of the oldest addictive substances known to man, is endemic all over the world except in Islamic countries where it is strictly banned by the *Koran*.[16] The French mathematician Sully Ledermann[17] was the first scientist to study the distribution of consumption of alcohol in different populations. These systematic surveys report the frequency and amount of alcohol consumption in the French population. He reported that the more consumers of alcohol there were in society, the more alcoholics and problems associated with alcoholism. This observation seems to derive from common sense, but Ledermann gave it a mathematical formulation which relates the number of "excessive" users of alcohol to the overall average consumption of all consumers. If mean consumption decreases by approximately one-half, excessive drinking will decrease by two-thirds. He reported that in France, which holds the world record of per capita consumption of alcohol, 7% to 9% of the consumers of alcohol drink excessively, which represents 2 million alcoholics, a staggering number when translated in premature death and disability. And this figure does not include the accidents caused by occasional acute intoxication, mainly road accidents. Ledermann concluded that in order to decrease the incidence of alcoholism and alcohol-related damage, one had to attempt to decrease the overall consumption of alcohol in the population. This conclusion was validated by the marked decrease in cases of alcoholic-induced liver cirrhosis or dementia observed in

France during the German occupation when alcoholic beverages were rationed and average consumption was drastically cut.

A similar analysis of "distribution of consumption" may be applied to the consumption of other dependence–producing drugs.[18] Surveys of cannabis consumption made in Jamaican villages, where the drug is freely available and socially acceptable, indicate that over 50% of the villagers who smoke marijuana consume it heavily every day: they smoke an equivalent of ten joints a day. In the United States, it has been found that among the population of high school seniors who reported smoking marijuana during 1978, 18% of them consumed the drug daily. We have seen that 90% of the Indians of the Andes who chew coca leaves consume them daily in thirty to fifty gram amounts equivalent to 300 to 500 mg. of cocaine base, a hefty dose.[19] And it is common knowledge that heroin users have to consume their drug of choice every day.

The results of these epidemiologic surveys indicate that in populations of drug consumers, the respective percentage of users which will become addicted is, to a major extent, related to the specific addictive property of the drug in the brain of the user. This addictive potential may be gauged by the incidence and rapidity of the development of compulsive drug–consuming in amounts damaging to health, after exposure to a given drug.

On the basis of epidemiologic surveys, which have been summarized above, the dependency producing potential of cannabis, and that of cocaine and heroin, would be, respectively, 7 and 14 times greater than the addictive potential of alcohol. It seems therefore fallacious to recommend the legalization model of alcohol as a solution to curtail the epidemic consumption of the illicit drugs which have much greater addictive properties.

The addictive power of cocaine and its epidemic spread are today apparent to all. The compulsive behavior of the pastaleros of Lima has been duplicated by the free basers and the crack smokers of American cities.

In New York City the epidemic spread of cocaine, between 1986 and 1988, mainly under the form of crack, is particularly illustrative. In the course of these three years, the number of cocaine users more than tripled from 182,000 to 600,000. Arrests for criminal offenses, mainly related to "crack," rose from 13,600 to 31,200; the city jail population increased from 10,000 to 18,000; there was a tripling of child abuse under drug influence from 2,600 to 8,200; the homicide rate rose by 10%; and crack played a role in 38% of the 1987 murders reported in 1988.[20]

Similar figures are surpassed only by those reported from Washington, D.C., which in 1988[21] became the capital murder city of the United States, with more homicides per capita than any other town in the country. Most of these crimes are related to cocaine traffic or consumption, and occur, as they do in New York, in the black and Hispanic ghettos of the inner city. In those areas the pervasive use of cocaine is threatening many of the hard-won social improvements achieved by the minorities over the past decade. It appears that cocaine is leading inner cities of the United States, including its capital, to the re-emergence of a two-tiered society.

In considering such facts one may wonder why prestigious opinion–makers are today still advocating the relegalization of cocaine sales; *The Economist,* one of the best informed and most influential weekly magazines in the western world, made this very recommendation editorially as late as January of 1989.[22] And in April of 1989 a group of academics from Princeton and Harvard, and Colombia, Venezuela, and Britain founded in Rome an International League Against Prohibition (of illicit drug use). The conference was hosted by the Italian Radical Party led by member of parliament, Marco Pannella, and already popularized by its lady representative Cicciolina, who does not hesitate to striptease in front of her audiences. The Italian Radical Party spent $200,000 of its government subsidy to organize the new league, which wants to promote across Western Europe a policy of legalization of the sale of illicit drugs, including heroin and cocaine. Mr. Pannella believes that such a policy should bring more votes to his party, greater visibility in Europe, and therefore larger subsidies in its coffers.[23] Such extreme manifestations should not be taken lightly in the present climate of cultural confusion prevailing in the West.[24] Rather than laugh about such a radical capitulation in the war on the cocaine epidemic, which is starting to invade Western Europe, it is time to define the solutions which will stop this scourge.

29

The Rehabilitation of the Cocaine Addict and the Will to Win the Cocaine Wars

The changes induced by cocaine in areas of the brain that regulate reward and memory, thereby affecting personality and survival, are foreboding; they are, in too many cases, irreversible. Man's future is threatened by this drug.

These stark observations must not be overlooked when one is referring to the treatment of the cocaine addict for whom there is no specific cure, as the early reformers, physicians or laymen, of the turn of the century had already emphasized. The outpatient treatment of addiction by purely pharmacological or psychological methods has yielded questionable results in spite of the remarkable achievements in most other areas of medicine. A fact that compounds this therapeutic uncertainty is that the addict rarely seeks "treatment" spontaneously because of his predicament, so well-described by the psychoanalyst Sandoz Rado.[1] The addict, says Rado, "does not suffer from his disease but enjoys it" and therefore has a great reluctance to be treated because treatment means he must give up his favorite reward and literally break up a love affair.

Attempts to treat heroin addiction with chemical substances such as methadone, naltrexone, or clonidine have been disappointing to the scientists and physicians who developed these treatment after painstaking efforts.[2] And yet they were based on the use of specific agents targeted to brain mechanisms which induce either euphoria or withdrawal symptoms. The suppression of the latter does not result in a cure, since a powerful dominant memory remains imprinted on the brain and orients the addict towards renewed drug taking. Furthermore, the medications which are used for the treatment of opiate withdrawal or for opiate maintenance are not effective in the case of cocaine addiction. The medications selected in our laboratory will alleviate only the acute toxic symptoms produced by this drug[3] and should be administered under medical supervision. Some investigators have attempted to alleviate cocaine withdrawal symptoms, depression and anxiety, by antidepressant medications, with uncertain outcome.[4] In any event, as was noted by Lewin and Maier, the dissipation of unpleasant withdrawal symptoms is a matter of days or weeks, and should not be construed as a "treatment" of cocaine addiction but as the first step towards total abstinence which may only be achieved through a long period of rehabilitation. To give up the drug, as Lewin declared nearly a century ago, "the cocaine addict must submit to at least one year of residence in a closed ward where he will learn how to live without the drug.[5] Such a rehabilitation implies a profound change in the way of life and the behavior of the addict who will have to resign himself to a disciplined existence.

Today, group living in specialized centers, or "therapeutic communities" ("T.C.'s," as they are called), offers the best chance of recovery for the cocaine addict. The goal of the T.C.'s is to restore the former addict to a drug-free existence, based on a socially productive life centered around family and community activities, very much like the model of the extended family pioneered with success by "Alcoholics Anonymous." Unlike the alcoholic who, after a three week "drying out" period in a specialized center, may return to his daily activities while following at the same time an outpatient, weekly program, the cocaine addict will have to remain as a resident in a therapeutic community for an extended period of time: one year or more. For heroin addicts, the first T.C. in the U.S. to adopt the concept of a rehabilitation with an extended family or the "family approach to recovery," as Monsignor O'Brien,[6] head of DayTop,[7] defines it, was Synanon during the great heroin epidemic of the sixties. The T.C.'s recruits are addicts who want to become drug–free and are not attracted by methadone maintenance; many of them have also experienced costly and limited periods of confinement in a psychiatric clinic for "treatment" of withdrawal symptoms, which were followed by a new bout of addiction.

Staffed in great part by recovered addicts, directed by dedicated leaders, the programs of the T.C.'s do represent a significant improvement over the detoxification regimens of the medical clinics. The T.C.'s have developed effective programs, unknown in the past, which offer a new hope for rehabilitation from addiction in the present era.

I had a chance to visit a number of them — the communities of DayTop Village created by Monsignor O'Brien in New York and California; Phoenix House T.C.'s[8] led by Dr. Mitchell Rosenthal; Kids of Bergen County,[9] directed by Dr. Miller Newton; the "Straight"[10] groups created in the eighties for teenagers — they all attest to the ever-increasing demand for such services which have not received the support that they deserve from the federal bureaucracy. In Europe the sixty T.C.'s of Le Patriarche Lucien Engelmayer, which started in France,[11] serve more than 3000 addicts undergoing rehabilitation. This list, far from complete, attests to the success of the T.C.'s in returning thousands of addicts to a drug free life.[12]

All therapeutic communities share the same general belief that a drug-free life brings about positive changes in a person and the rediscovery of a "joie de vivre" which has been called by Lucien Engelmayer, "the dynamics of rehabilitation." The T.C.'s differ according to their leadership, their recruits, and their staffing, but they all share similar guidelines which their residents must live by and which are: a total abstinence from all dependency-causing drugs, including alcohol but excluding tobacco and coffee; the acceptance of rules of communal living with all of its daily responsibilities of housekeeping chores; and participation in cultural, physical, and intellectual activities to prepare for a useful re-insertion into society. Such programs are aimed at a physical and mental reconditioning of body and brain so that natural, healthy activities may take precedence again and confer on the individual a good measure of satisfaction and self-esteem.

T.C.'s are often run by educators or clerics with no medical or psychiatric training, assisted by recovered addicts. The cost of residence is moderate. This type of organization has generated some controversy between rehabilitation communities and more expensive hospital-based programs staffed by health professionals.

The population of the T.C.'s has changed from a predominance of heroin addicts in the sixties and seventies to one of cocaine addicts since the mid-eighties.

In terms of overall rehabilitative goals, as documented by

Professor deLeon,[13] the T.C. is effective especially for those who remain beyond a year in residence. After one year spent in a T.C. the former addict has one chance in two to lead a drug-free, socially useful life. A national survey performed in 1981 showed that 37% of former T.C. residents were drug-free and employed two years after they had left the community. These statistics show some improvement over those from the Lexington narcotic "farm" in Kentucky where incarcerated convicted addicts were treated in the late thirties. There the relapse rate exceeded 80% one year after the release of the former addicts from prison.

Rehabilitation, however effective it may be, is not a cure for drug dependence. Lasting behavioral change is dependent on other factors related in great part to the social milieu which determines drug availability and acceptability. As long as the social climate condones or promotes drug use, such as alcohol, marijuana, and cocaine, rehabilitation and the efforts of the addict striving for a drug-free life will be weakened. Rehabilitated addicts must adjust to a society still profoundly influenced by the need for chemical gratification and by the all-pervasive message of the drug culture extolling the joys of altered consciousness. Conversely, according to Professor deLeon, coercion in treatment through rational or legal pressure often leads drug abusers to rehabilitation. These factors lead to increased retention time in the T.C. which is in turn related to long-term success.

However, rehabilitation alone will not curtail an epidemic of drug addiction. "Indeed," writes Bejerot, "only a minority of drug addicts will spontaneously enlist in a treatment center, and if they do so, it usually is four to five years after they started drug self-administration."[14] "Treatment" or "rehabilitation" of the addict is not a substitute for general interdiction measures, which have been successfully applied in other countries or in other times.

We have already reported the Japanese and Chinese examples which prove the effectiveness of interdiction measures in controlling drug addiction when there exists a national consensus on the refusal of recreational drug use. Because of their severity, they may not be applicable to countries which are less structured and disciplined than Japan and China.

More recently, the Republic of Singapore has succeeded in controlling an epidemic of heroin in its most addictive form:

the inhaling of the blue cloud of smoke from the burning powder, a custom which is called "chasing the dragon." The addiction control model used in Singapore is less drastic than that in Japan. While the repression of supply is pitiless, the measures taken to decrease the demand for heroin apply on a large scale the methods used in the therapeutic communities but on a coercive basis. In 1985 I visited Singapore[15] (population 2.2 million), an island close to a sea of opium poppies produced in the nearby Golden Triangle. In 1977, the number of heroin sniffers (who require triple the dosage of intravenous users) was estimated at 13,000, up from a few hundred in 1973, and an estimated 3% of males aged 15–24 were involved, threatening the economic development of the island.

Poh Geok Ek, head of the Central Narcotics Bureau, recalls: "The situation called for immediate action; otherwise heroin, like an infectious disease, would spread like wildfire. We found to our dismay that countries in the west from which we learned advanced technology had failed to curb the drug problem. Some even advocate giving heroin to the addicts." From Mr. Poh's reactions, I could see that this so called "British model" revived the stinging memory of the Opium Wars.

"Supply reduction was based on adopting the death penalty for trafficking in more than 15 grams (0.425 ounce) of pure heroin. Fifteen persons have been hanged in the past five years, over 2,000 traffickers were arrested, and many were retained in 'preventive detention.' However, our major effort was directed at demand reduction," Mr. Poh said.

Operation Ferret began in 1977 with the large–scale arrest of suspected users and (after a positive urine sample) their immediate commitment, without court proceedings, to drug rehabilitation centers (DRC's).

Mr. Poh describes the program as follows: "After withdrawal without supportive medication (cold turkey), the detainees undergo a six-month to one-year program aimed at instilling discipline, social responsibility, and sound work habits. Our aim is to persuade the addict that he no longer needs the drug and finally to give him an incentive to replace the drug with a more satisfying way of life. Activities in DRC's are devoted first to indoctrination and a military-type program of exercise and calisthenics, followed by employment in industrial workshops."

This period is followed by six months in a "day release scheme" or halfway house to provide gradual adjustment to a free environment. After completion of this period, the released inmate is placed on a 24-month drug supervision program that requires weekly to monthly urinalysis. Counseling is provided by volunteers.

Through Operation Ferret the estimated number of heroin addicts was reduced to 6,000 in 1983 from 13,000 in 1977, and the number of new addicts detected per month decreased to 59 from 573. The street price of heroin rose from $35 to $400 per gram, despite bumper harvests in the nearby Golden Triangle. The relapse rate, after release from the centers, fell from 70% in 1979 to 42% in 1983.

"The cost is high," says Mr. Poh. "[Some] $2.5 million for enforcement and $11.5 million for treatment and rehabilitation. But it has rapid dividends."

The success of China, Japan, and Singapore in their fight against drug addiction is linked to their compliance with a philosophy which stresses the necessity of maintaining the natural balance of the mind, expressed in the teachings of Confucius, Lao Tse, and Buddha, who counseled his followers: "You will refuse any substance that intoxicates the mind." A respect for reason and moderation is just as much part of our Western culture, since it has inspired so many individuals to think freely and rationally while repudiating the poisons of the brain.

This rule to safeguard our spirit has been handed down to us through the centuries in Biblical texts that shaped our history. Breaking away from the Greco-Roman cult of Dionysius and Bacchus, Saint Paul warns his disciples against excessive libation conducive to loud and boisterous behavior inconsistent with joyous Christian conviviality. Addressing the Corinthians, he cautions them against intoxication with wine, although this beverage is a symbol of the New Alliance.[16] And Saint Paul reminds his flock that "the drunken will not know the Kingdom of God" because they have lost their free will and their ability to recognize all that is holy. Many centuries before and ever since, the Hebrews preached and practiced sobriety, respectful of the warnings of the Old Testament "that the fathers have eaten sour grapes and the children's teeth are set on edge."[17] These words have inspired many physicians throughout the centuries, and have supported the art of healing.

The medical arts, ever since the remote ages of Imenhotep[18] and Hippocrates,[19] have strived to heal by assisting mother nature in restoring the normal balance of body regulations impaired by disease. Ambroise Paré, a sixteenth century surgeon who discovered how to tie off blood vessels to control bleeding during amputations, instead of using cauterization, declared simply: "I treat my patients; God heals them." Paré called on God to explain the miracle of natural regulations that restore the inherent balance of body function and with it, physical and mental health.[20] Today's rehabilitation communities are inspired by the same conviction that will help liberate the brain of an addict from the clutches of drugs and restore his will to live as a free person.

In this context the magic pharmacological bullet sought by some scientists and psychiatrists to cure addiction appears as a remote pipe dream; such a drug would endow healers with the infinite power of chemically restoring the equilibrium and integrity of brain mechanisms which control reason and free will.

Science can supply us with the physiological basis for rejecting the recreational use of cocaine and other substances which alter the internal milieu of the brain and impair its function. What is needed is the will to implement this knowledge into action — a step which will ensure the continuity and survival of our culture and history.

The study of life sciences has constantly reaffirmed Claude Bernard's basic principle that stresses the necessity of maintaining a stable internal environment in order to secure a free life.[21] But a scientific principle by itself does not carry the power that will motivate human behavior. The French physician and author Rabelais[22] put it well 500 years ago in his aphorism: "Science without conscience is but the ruination of the soul."

Another physician might have endowed Bernard's definition of life with the dynamic thrust liable to rally hearts and minds: Albert Schweitzer, the Renaissance man of our century — theologian, musician, and Christian missionary.[23]

I found this out some thirty years ago, when my wife and I visited the "great white doctor" in his Alsatian retreat of

Gunsbach where he was vacationing. After playing a Bach fugue on the old "piano organ" he had received from the Bach Society in 1912, Albert Schweitzer chatted with us, recalling his life in Gabon, at Lambarene, in the brush hospital he had built with his own hands at the edge of the jungle. "One evening, while I was rowing down the Ogowe after visiting a patient, a thought flashed through my mind: Reverence for life."

"It happened like that, suddenly?" I asked him.

"Yes, just like that, all of a sudden. But I had been thinking about it for quite a long time." He smiled and looked at us, his deep blue eyes twinkling with humor.

"You see," he went on, "I'm also an heir to the Aufklarung, the age of Enlightenment and of Reason!"

By referring to reverence for life and the exercise of Reason, Albert Schweitzer had brought together the joint messages from the heart and the intelligence, sprung from the vital sources of our Western civilization and endowed with universal value. They will continue to hearten all those who are committed to the fight that will, in the long run, win the cocaine wars in order to ensure the safeguard of man.

Victory will be achieved by winning the battle of the mind, so clearly defined in the preamble of the charter of UNESCO, the cultural organization of the United Nations. "Since war starts in the mind of men it is in the mind of men that it has to be fought." Such a metaphor illustrates the importance of fighting the erroneous ideas, prejudices, and ignorance which generate major conflicts throughout the world, including the drug wars.

The battle ahead of us will be primarily one of the mind and waged on two fronts. It will have to rebut the arguments of the modern sophists who wish to turn the clock back and relegalize all addictive drugs by propagating pseudo-scientific rhetoric and social nihilism. And, foremost, it will uphold the rules which have to be accepted by citizens of a progressive society dedicated "to freedom under the law."

The restoration of a national consensus to refuse the "recreational" or "responsible" use of addictive drugs will be a most difficult task in the United States. It will require the support of the mass media which in the past two decades have sent billions of pervasive and ambiguous messages which condoned or tolerated illicit drug use, or at best adopted a neutral stand. In order to stop the great white plague, the mass media, television, film, and press will have to start exerting, as they did in the past, a measure of restraint, and adopt towards illicit drug use a stand, at least as negative as the stand displayed against tobacco smoking or pollution of the environment. The glamorous and fashionable aspects of drug taking should no longer be favorably exposed on the movie or TV screen. Opinions of civil libertarians concerning the relegalization of illicit drugs, even when editorially expounded, should be matched by rebuttals of equal length, as exemplified by veteran *New York Times* editorialist A. M. Rosenthol.[24]

Americans will be motivated by the pioneering examples of Theodore Roosevelt and the Progressive Movement who were able to check the opium epidemic which was prevailing at the turn of the century in China and, to a lesser extent, in the United States. These historical examples will be duplicated when the same political determination of the American people is revived.

Supply reduction will require national and international interdiction measures. The gradual eradication of coca-bush plantations must be initiated in the producing countries, together with a program for planting basic food crops and training the local peasantry in modern farming techniques. Such a scheme calls for a new multi-billion-dollar, ecologically sound United Nations assistance program (with the cooperation and contribution of the USSR) staggered over many years. An international task force may be required to control illicit traffic.

At the same time, the consuming country must lower its demand by more strictly enforcing existing laws that ban use and possession of cocaine. Dealers should be subjected to the same sentences imposed on murderers. Confirmed drug addicts must accept society's decision to be responsible for rehabilitating them to a drug-free life, after they have been clearly identified. This should require systematic testing and compulsory treatment and rehabilitation.

Such measures rely upon a strongly-expressed sentiment of societal disapproval of cocaine and other illicit drug use by all segments of society. Interdiction measures cannot be effective in a climate of cultural and media acceptance of "recreational" drug use. Only when the vital grass roots of America, feeling their existence threatened, as after Pearl Harbor, become really determined to fight drugs, will they be capable of waging a war, with their allies, until victory is achieved.

At the end of the 20th century, the leaders of the United States and the USSR are taking bold steps to lessen and in the long run eliminate the threat of a global atomic war which could destroy half the planet. Their next endeavor will be to eliminate the scourge of widespread availability and trivialization of mind-enslaving drugs which threaten our children, the wave of the future. The United States of America, as it did at the turn of the century, should again lead the way to reach this challenging goal.[25]

Notes for the Curious Reader

Chapter 1   Farid at the Hotel Pierre

1. C. V. Wetli and R. K. Wright, "Death Caused by Recreational Cocaine Use" (*Journal of the American Medical Association* 241 (1979): 1519–22).
2. Hans Wolfgang Maier (1882–1945). Originally published in 1926 as *Der Kokainismus — Geschichte/Pathologie Medizinische und Behordliche Bekampfung* (Leipzig: George Thieme Verlag). It was translated into French by Dr. S. Jankelevitch (*La Cocaïne — Historique — Pathologique — Clinique — Thérapeutique — Défense Sociale* (Paris: Payot, 1928); and into English by Oriana Josseau Kalant for the Alcoholism and Drug Addiction Research Foundation (Toronto, 1987). It is this English edition to which we refer in our notes, hereinafter cited as "H. Maier, *Der Kokainismus.*"
3. L. Natansohn and L. Lipskeroff, "Uber Perforation der Knorpeligen Nasenscheiderwand bei Kokainschnupfern" (Z. Hals-, Nasen-, Ohrenhlk, 7:409, 1924). Leon Natansohn was a Russian physician who examined ninety-eight heavy cocaine users in a Moscow clinic in 1920. He found that eighty-four of them had a perforated septum.
4. L. D. Johnston, J. G. Balchman, and P. M. O'Malley, "Highlights from Student Drug Use in America, 1975–1980" (Washington, D.C.: Department of Health and Human Services Publication No. (ADM) 81–1066, U. S. Government Printing Office, 1980).

Chapter 2   A Chewed-Up Nose

1. Wetli and Wright, pp. 2519–22.

Chapter 3   From Cocaine to Vitamins

1. Lucien Engelmayer, called "The Patriarche" because of his long white beard, is the founder and director of the "Association Le Patriarche," the largest rehabilitation drug-free organization in France and Spain. The organization is not unlike DayTop or Phoenix House in the United States.

Chapter 4   The Curtain Falls

1. The French criminal code has a section which provides a fine and imprisonment for "anyone who does not assist a person whose life is in danger."

Chapter 5   A Trial in Newark and Cement Boots

1. G. G. Nahas, "A Pharmacological Classification of Drug Abuse" (*Bulletin of Narcotics* 33, No. 2 (1981): 1–19). The author describes cocaine as an addictive drug which is self-administered and induces tolerance as well as withdrawal symptoms.
2. Lester Grinspoon in "Hearings on the Health Consequences of Marijuana Use" (Washington, D.C.: Committee on the Judiciary of the United States, January 16–18, 1980 (Serial No. 96–54), U.S. Government Printing Office, pp. 30–35). Dr. Grinspoon's testimony summarizes the conclusion of his book, *Marijuana Reconsidered* (Cambridge, MA: Harvard University Press, 1971).
3. Lester Grinspoon and J. P. Bakalar, *Cocaine* (New York: Plenum Press, 1975, pp. 1–308).
4. Amphetamines are synthetic compounds which have psychostimulant properties similar to those of cocaine.
5. Barbiturates are sleeping pills which, when taken regularly, produce tolerance. Cessation of their chronic use induces withdrawal symptoms which may be life-threatening.
6. "L.S.D." stands for Lysergic Acid Diethylamide, a powerful synthetic hallucinogen.
7. In his paper, "Toxic Effects Folowing the Use of Local Anesthetics," Emil Mayer reports twenty-six deaths due to

the application of cocaine solution during surgical procedures. (*Journal of the American Medical Association* 82 (1924): 876–85.)

8. This film is available from the University of Michigan Audiovisual Department. It is described by G. Deneau, T. Yanagita, and M. H. Seevers in "Self-Administration of Psychoactive Substances by the Monkey" (*Psychopharmacologia* 16 (1969): 30–48).

9. Grinspoon and Bakalar, "A Kick from Cocaine" (*Psychology Today* 10 (1977): 41–2).

10. Norman E. Zinberg and John A. Robertson, *Drugs and the Public* (New York: Simon and Schuster, 1972).

11. A. T. Weil, "Why Coca Leaf Should be Available as a Recreational Drug" (*Journal of Psychedelic Drugs* 9 (1977): 75–8).

12. Testimony of Dr. Charles Schuster in *People of State of Illinois v. Thomas Santori, et al.* (March 2, 1981). In this court case, the defense successfully challenged the constitutionality of the classification of cocaine as a narcotic drug. This classification was claimed to be "violative of equal protection." The court agreed, stating that "cocaine is a stimulant, not a narcotic, and unlike the opiates it does not induce tolerance or withdrawal symptoms. . . . There is no causal connection between ingestion of cocaine and criminal behavior. . . . It is the consensus within the scientific and medical community that cocaine is a drug with low abuse potential and not very dangerous." However, the court rejected the demand for changing the schedule of cocaine classification and ordered that it remain in Schedule II because "though cocaine is the least dangerous drug in this Schedule, its potential for abuse is much greater than that of Schedule III substances." On the basis of the scientific evidence presented by Dr. Ronald Siegel, this judgment has the wisdom of Solomon.

13. See Dr. Schuster's testimony in the *Thomas Santori* case.

14. The New Testament (King James Version), Matthew 7:1.

15. *The Cocaine Papers,* edited by Robert Byck, M.D. (New York: Stonehill, 1974). The book is the most complete reference, in an English translation, on the subject of Freud's work on cocaine. It includes Freud's letters, his papers, and his dreams, as well as passages from the work of Freud's biographer, Ernest Jones.

16. L. Lewin, *Phantastica: Narcotic and Stimulant Drugs,* translated from the second German edition by P. H. A. Wirth (New York: Dutton, 1931; French translation, Paris: Payot, 1928).
17. H. Maier, *Der Kokainismus.*

Chapter 6   Freud's Praise of Cocaine

1. Albert Nieman, *Uber eine neue Base in den Kokablattern in Dissertation* (Gottingen: 1860).
2. Wilhelm Lossen, "Uber das Kokain" (*Ann. Chem. Pharm.,* 1865).
3. T. Aschenbrandt, "Die physiologische Wirkung und Bedeutung des Cocain. Muriat auf den menschlichen Organismus" (*Dtsch. Med. Wochenschr.* 9 (1883): 730).
4. *Cocaine Papers,* ed. R. Byck.
5. Sigmund Freud, "Uber Coca" (*Wiener Zentralblatt fur die gesamte Therapie* 2 (1884): 289–314). Reprinted in Byck's edition of *Cocaine Papers.*
6. Antoine Laurent Jussieu (1748–1863). French botanist. He expanded the national system of plant classification formulated by his uncle Bernard (1744–1829).
7. Jean Baptiste Pierre de Monet Lamarck (1744–1829). French naturalist. Among his publications was a dictionary of botany, *Encyclopédie Méthodique Botanique* (1783–1796).
8. For an historical account of coca cultivation and use under the Incas, see Remedio de la Pena Bengue, "El Uso de la Coca entre las Incas" (*Revista Española de Antropologica Americana* 79 (1972): 277–304); Carlos Gutierrez-Noriega, "El Cocaismo y la Alimentación en el Peru" (*Anales de la Facultad de Medicina* 31 (1948): 1–90); and W. Golden Mortimer, *Peru, History of Coca* (New York: J. A. Vail, 1901, reprinted Berkeley, CA: And/Or Press, 1974).
9. De la Pena Bengue; Gutierrez-Noriega; and Mortimer.
10. Johann Jakob von Tschudi, German archaeologist and explorer. He visited Peru about 1833 and was most impressed by the stimulatory properties of cocaine, which he reported in his *Memoires.*
11. Edward Poeppig, German physician. He visited Peru in 1836 and was highly critical of coca in his memoirs. He claims that "the coca leaf chewer is a slave of his passion

even more than a drunk, is incapable of pursuing serious goals in life, is a victim of anemia, digestive troubles, and hallucinations" (quoted in Maier, *Der Kokainismus*).

12. Antonio de Julian, a Jesuit priest who visited Peru in the late 18th century. In 1787 he suggested that coca be substituted for tea. He is quoted in H. Maier, *Der Kokainismus*.

13. Nicolas Monardes, Spanish physician. He was the first to describe, in 1580, the features and virtues of the coca plant, along with those of other herbs and trees. He is quoted in H. Maier, *Der Kokainismus*.

14. Claude Bernard (1813–1873). French physician and the founder of physiology as an exact science. In his classic treatise, *Introduction a l'Étude de la Médecine Expérimentale* (1865) he laid the foundations of the experimental method in physiology. He held that body mechanisms strive to maintain a constant inner environment ("milieu interieur") through self-regulation. To achieve this equilibrium the various physiological and biochemical processes of the body have to be under an integrated (cerebral) control.

15. Claude Bernard, *Leçons de Pathologie Experimentale* (1872). This same experiment was also duplicated by the Russian physiologist Vassili von Anrep ("Uber die physiologische Wirkung des Cocaine," *Pflugers Arch. ges. Physiol. Mensch, Tiere* 21 (1860): 38).

16. *Morena y Mais* (Paris: T. Thesis, 1868). This anecdote was reported by a Peruvian physician, Hipolete Unanue.

17. Paolo Mantegazza, an Italian neurologist who was very influential in the late 19th century. His autiobiographical essay on cocaine was extremely popular (*Sulle virtu ingieniche e medicinali della coca*, Milan: Autosservazione, 1959).

18. Karl Schroff, "Vorlaufige Mitteilung über Kokain" (*Wiender Medizinische Wochenschrift* 34, 1862).

19. See note 15.

20. See not 17.

21. René Descartes (1596–1650). French mathematician and philosopher. He laid the foundations of modern geometry and algebra. As a philosopher, he made a radical distinction between mind and matter.

Chapter 7   Cocaine as a Cure for Morphine Addiction: Freud's "Parapraxis"

1. Between 1880 and 1884 the *Detroit Therapeutic Gazette* published sixteen reports of the cure of the opium habit by coca. The first was by W. H. Bentley (*Detroit Therapeutic Gazette* 4 (1880): 253-4); also an editorial on the subject, p. 172 of the same issue). Bentley, who admitted using coca since 1870, claimed it cured impotence and that it was a drug of choice in health and disease. By 1883 the American pharmaceutical company Parke Davis had marketed cocaine and advertised it in its medical journals for the treatment of morphine addiction and alcoholism. Besides these indications, cocaine was recommended for many other ailments, which were subsequently described by Freud in *Uber Coca*.
2. Marxow Ernest von Fleishl, a physiologist in the faculty of the Vienna Medical School and a close friend of Freud.
3. *St. Louis Medical Journal,* June 1886.
4. Charles Fauvel, in *The Efficacy of Coca Erythoxylon: Notes and Comments by Prominent Physicians,* 2d. ed. (New York and Paris: Mariani and Company, 1888).
5. K. Koller, "Uber die Verwendung des Kokains zur Anasthesierung am Auge" (*Wiener Medizinische Wochenschrift* 34 (1884): 1276-1309). For the story of Koller's discovery see Hortense Koller Becker, "Carl Koller and Cocaine," in *Psychoanalytic Quarterly* 32 (1962): 309-73.
6. Jean Martin Charcot (1825-1893). French physician. He developed in the Salpétrière Hospital of Paris, the greatest clinic of his time for diseases of the nervous system. He was one of the founders of the science of neurology. Using hypnotism, he investigated the nature of hysteria, which led Freud to his early formulation of the psychoanalytic theory to account for this disease.
7. Freud, "Uber Coca" (*Wiener Therapie*), pp. 289-98. (Vienna: Vienna, 1885).
8. Sigmund Freud, "Beitrag zur Kenntnis der Cocawirkung" (*Wiener Medizinische Wochenschrift* 35 (1885): 129-33, reprinted in *Cocaine Papers,* pp. 97-104, as "Contribution to the Knowledge of the Effect of Cocaine").
9. Albrecht Erlenmeyer, "Uber die Wirkung des Kokains bei der Morphiumentziehung" (*Zentralblatt fur Nervhk. Psych. u. gerichtl. Psychopath* 8 (1885): 289-93).
10. Sigmund Freud, "Bermerkunger über Kokainsucht und Kokainfurcht" (*Wiener Medizinische Wochenschrift* 28 (1887):

929–932, reprinted in *Cocaine Papers* at pp. 171–6 as "Craving for and Fear of Cocaine").

11. W. A. Hammond, "Remarks on Cocaine and the So-called Cocaine Habit" (*Journal of Nervous Mental Disorders* 11 (1886): 754–58).

12. W. A. Hammond, "Coca: Its Preparations and Their Therapeutical Qualities, with Some Remarks on the So-called 'Cocaine Habit' " (*Transactions of the Medical Society of Virginia* 10 (1887): 215–19).

13. William Steward Halsted (1852–1922). The use of cocaine by this most prominent American surgeon led to his temporary disability, which required hospitalizations and a year's cruise to the Caribbean. After his rehabilitation from cocaine addiction he returned to a productive and brilliant career. He remained addicted to morphine, however, as revealed by his colleague, Sir William Osler, who is quoted in the history of Halsted's life written by his pupil, the neurosurgeon Wilder Penfield, in "Halsted of Johns Hopkins" (*Journal of the American Medical Association* 210 (1969): 2214–18). Halsted's life has also been detailed by J. I. Ingle, "William Halsted, Pioneer in Oral Nerve Block Injection and Victim of Drug Experimentation" (*Journal of the American Dental Association* 82 (1971): 46–7).

14. D. P. Ausubel, *Drug Addiction: Physiological, Psychological and Sociological Aspects* (New York: Random House, 1958, pp. 43–4). The addiction-prone theory of drug addiction has never been supported by psychometric studies of addicts. See P. and L. P. Gendreau, "Addiction Prone Personality: A Study of Canadian Heroin Addicts," in *Classical Contributions in the Addictions,* ed. Howard Shaffer and Milton Earl Burglass (New York: Bruner/Mazel, 1981).

15. H. Maier, *Der Kokainismus.*

16. Ernest Jones, *The life and Work of Sigmund Freud,* Vol. 2 (New York: Basic Books, 1953), p. 189.

17. Ibid.

18. Claude Olivenstein, "Evolution de la Toxicothérapie depuis dix ans" (in *Drogue et Civilisation,* ed. G. Nahas (Paris: Pergamon Press 1982), p. 104).

19. Sigmund Freud, *Das Unbehagen in Der Kultur* (Vienna Internationaler Psychoanlytischer Verlag). There is a translation of the pertinent passage by J. Strachey on page 25 of *Civilization and its Discontents* (New York: Norton, 1961).

20. Jurgen von Scheidt, "Sigmund Freud und das Kokain" (*Psyche* 27 (1973).

21. *Ibid.*

22. Lester Grinspoon and J. P. Bakalar, *Cocaine,* pp. 1–36.

23. E. M. Thornton, *Freud and Cocaine — the Freudian Fallacy* (London: Blond & Briggs, 1983).

24. H. Eysenck, *Decline and Fall of the Freudian Empire* (New York: Viking Books, 1985), chapter viii.

Chapter 8   Erlenmeyer and Lewin's Indictment of Cocaine:
            God is a Substance

1. Albrecht Erlenmeyer (1822–1899). Pioneering German psychiatrist. He dominated the field in Germany, where he created a large psychiatric hospital for brain and nervous disorders and special establishments for mentally retarded patients. He carried out research on statistics of mental illness and morphine addiction and published numerous papers. He was an advocate of the somatic (organic) school of mental illness and of close connection between psychiatry and neurology.

2. A. Erlenmeyer, "Uber Kokainsucht" (*Dtsch. Med.-Ztg.* 7:483, 1886), and, by the same author, "Uber die Wirkung des Kokains bei der Morphiumentziehung (*Zentralblatt für Nervhk. Psych. u. Gerichtl. Psychopath.* 8: 289, 1985).

3. A. Erlenmeyer, *Die Morphiumensucht und ihre Behandlung,* 3rd edition (Berlin: Heusser, 1887), p. 154.

4. Ludwig Lewin (1859–1929), German physician, the founder of modern toxicology. For bibliographical details see Bo Holmsted in *Phantastica,* pp. ix–xiv. In concluding Lewin's obituary, one of his pupils wrote: "Pharmacologist, toxicologist, medical historian, keen scientist, brilliant teacher, profound scholar, fascinating writer, a man of noble character, lofty ideals, and loyal to his race and faith."

5. Ludwig Lewin, *Nebenwirkungen der Arzneimittel, Pharmakologish. klin. Handbook* (Berlin: A. Hirschwald 1897).

6. Ludwig Lewin, *Besl. Klein Wochenschrift* 8 (1885): 326–28).

7. Ludwig Lewin, *Die Gifte in der Weltgeschichte* (Berlin: Springer, 1920).

8. Ludwig Lewin, "Phantastica," in *Narcotic and Stimulating*

Drugs, Their Use and Abuse, translated by P. H. A. Wirth (London: Routledge & Kegan Paul, 1964; and New York: E. P. Dutton and Co., 1964, pp. 75–88).

9. Francisco Pizarro (1470–1541). Spanish conqueror of Peru.

10. The Second Council of Lima (Peru) in 1552 gathered lay and religious Spanish leaders.

11. Francisco de Toledo, Governor of Peru from 1560 to 1569.

12. Bo Holmsted in "Phantastica," p. x (American edition translated by E. P. Dutton).

13. Sigmund Freud, *Die Zunkunft einer Illusion* (Vienna: Internationale Psychanlytischer Verlag, 1927). James Strachey made an English translation, *The Future of an Illusion* (New York: Norton, 1961).

Chapter 9   Hans Maier and the Great Cocaine Epidemic at the Turn of the Century

1. From July to December, 1885, there were twenty-seven articles, notes, and letters on cocaine in the *New York Medical Journal.* They all recommended the drug for any of these conditions.

2. *Coca Erythoxylon and its Derivatives* (1887), a 101-page illustrated pamphlet by the Parke Davis Company, Detroit and New York.

3. Angelo Mariani and Company published many pamphlets which were widely distributed to pharmacists and physicians. They included *Coca and its Therapeutic Applications,* 1896; *The Effects of Coca Erythoxylon,* 1888; and *Mariani's Coca Leaf,* 1905.

4. E. J. Kahn, *The Big Drink: The Story of Coca Cola* (New York: Random House, 1960).

5. F. W. Ring, "Cocaine and Its Fascinations from a Personal Experience" (*Med. Record.* 32 (1887): 274–276).

6. *New York Medical Record,* May 29, 1886, quoted in H. Maier, *Der Kokainismus,* p. 26.

7. D. R. Brower, "Insanity from Cocaine" (*Journal of the American Medical Association,* 1886).

8. D. R. Brower, "The Effects of Cocaine on the Central Nervous System" (*Philadelphia Med. Surg. Reporter,* 1876).

9. T. D. Crothers, "Cocaine Inebriety" (*Med. Rec.* (New York) 77 (1910): 744).

10. *Ibid.*

11. G. W. Norris, "A Case of Cocaine Habit of Three Months' Duration, Treated by Complete and Immediate Withdrawal of the Drug" (*Philadelphia Medical Journal* 1 (1901): 304).

12. Penfield, pp. 2214–18, and Ingle, pp. 46–7.

13. T. G. Simonton, "The Increase of the Use of Cocaine among the Laity in Pittsburgh" (*Philadelphia Medical Journal* 11 (1903): 556).

14. L. Kolb and A. G. DuMez, "The Prevalence and Trend of Drug Addiction in the United States and Factors Influencing It" (*Public Health Report* 39 (1924): 1179).

15. M. J. Wilbert and M. G. Motter. *Digest of Laws and Regulations in Force in the United States Relating to the Possession, Use, Sale and Manufacture of Poisons and Habit-Forming Drugs* (Washington, D.C.: U.S. Treasury Department, 1912). These figures as well as those of Kolb and DuMez have been disputed by Alfred Lindesmith and other new reformers. However, statistics show that cocaine imports between 1898 and 1902 increased by 40% while the population had increased by only 10%.

16. A. Flexner, "Medical Education in the United States and Canada" (New York: Carnegie Foundation for the Advancement of Teaching Bulletin no. 4, 1910). This report recommended closure of substandard medical schools and gave the Johns Hopkins Medical School in Baltimore as a model modern medical school.

17. H. Maier, *Der Kokainismus.*

18. V. Magnan and L. Saury, "Trois Cas de Cocaïnisme Chronique" (Paris: Compt. Rend. Soc. Biol., (1889) 1: 60–3).

19. G. Guillain, "L'intoxication par la Cocaïne" (*Journal Medical Français* 7 (1914): 235).

20. H. Obersteiner, *Zur Internen Anwendung des Kokains bei Neurosen und Psychosen* (Vienna: Wien Med. Presse 26 (1885), p. 1253). By the same author: "Uber Intoxikationspsychosen (*Mitt. Wien. Med. Doct. Coll.* 12 (1886): 42). See also W. Ihlow, "Uber Morphio-Cocain-Paranoia" (Dissertation) (*Wien Klin.* 12 (1886): 33 and Berlin: G. Schade, 1895). Other references are: P. Schroder, "Intoxikations

psychosen," in *Aschaffenburg's Handbuch der Psychiatrie,* Section III, Part I (Leipzig and Vienna: Deuticke, 1912); J. Scherer, "Zur Kasuistik der Kokainspsychosen," in *Extracts from the Dissertations in the Faculty of Medicine, University of Cologne, 1919/20,* ed. A. Dietrich (Bonn: Marcus & Weber, 1921); E. Joel and F. Frankel, "Der Kokainismus: Ein Beitrag zur Geschichte und Psychopathologie der Rauschgifte" *(Erbeg. inn. Med. Kinderheilkd.* 25 (1924): 988).

21. R. Bucelli, "Cocainismo e delirio cocainico" *(Riv. Sper. Freniat.* 20 (1894): 69); S. Tomasini, "Sulla Psicosi Cocainica *(Il Manicomio* 20 (1904): 67; R. Romanese, "Osservazioni Medico-legali sopra un Avvelenamento Acuto da Cocaina" *(Riv. Med. Legale* (Pisa) 10 (1920): 39); F. Sabatucci, "Sindromi Neuropsichiche nei Fiutatori di Cocaina" *(Policlinico* (Rome) (Sez. Med.) 29: (1922): 235).

22. L. Saury, " 'Du Cocaïnisme. Contribution à L'étude du foli-toxique.' " *(Ann. Méd.-Psychol.,* Ser. 7, 9: (1889): 439). Also see P. Sollier, "Un Cas Remarquable de Cocaïnomanie" *(J. Méd. Paris* 22 (1910): 40); C. Vallon and R. Bessière, "Les Troubles Mentaux d'Origine Cocaïnique" *(Encéphale. J. Méd. Int.* (Paris) 18 (1914): 72); H. Piouffle, *Les Psychoses Cocaïniques* (Paris: A. Maloine et Fils, 1919); G. Guillain, *Etudes Neurologiques* (Paris: Masson & Cie., 1922).

23. A. Stein, "Ein Fall von Kokainvergiftung" *(Prag. Med. Wochenschr.,* 1904).

24. F. Lubet-Barbon, "Cocaïnisme Nasal" (Société de Laryngologie de Paris, February 18, 1908).

25. L. Natansohn and L. Lipskeroff, "Uber Perforation der knorpeligen Nasenscheiderwand bei Kokainschnupfern (Z. Hals-, Nasen-, Ohrenhlk, 7 (1924): 409).

26. H. Schnyder, "Ein Vall von Cocainvergiftung" *(Corr.-Bl. Schweiz. Aerzte* 17 (1887): 161).

27. E. Falke, "Nebenwirkungen von Intoxikationen bei der Anwendung neuerer Arzneimittel" *(Therap. Montash.,* 1890).

28. R. G. Smart and L. Anglin, "Do We Know the Lethal Dose of Cocaine?" *(Journal of Forensic Science* 32 (1987): 303–12).

29. A. Hautant, "Uber den Chronischen Kokainismus mit Nasaler Anwendung" *(Int. Zentralblatt Laryngol. Rhinol.* 25 (1909): 138).

30. K. Heilbronner, "Kokainpsychose" (*Z. ges. Neurol. Psychiat.* 15 (1913): 415).

31. H. Higier, "Beitrag zur Klinik der psychischen Storungen bei chronischem Kokainismus" (*Munch. med. Wochenschr.* 58 (1911): 503).

32. H. Maier, *Der Kokainismus,* pp. 145–216.

33. W. Straub, "Uber Kokainismus" (*Franfurter Zeitung,* Number 462, 25 April 1919).

34. E. Bravetta and G. Invernizzi, "Il Cocainismo: Osservazione cliniche Ricerche sperimentali e anatomopatologiche" (*Note Riv. Psichiatr.* 10 (1922): 543 and 11 (1923): 179).

35. G. G. Nahas, R. Trouvé, and M. Maillet, "Prevention of the Cardiotoxicity of Cocaine by Nitrendipine, a CA2+ Blocker" (*Bulletin Academie Nationale Médécine* 169 (1985): 1151–6.)

36. H. Maier, *Der Kokainismus,* p. 82.

37. *Ibid.,* p. 228.

38. *Ibid.,* pp. 82–90.

39. E. Joel and F. Frankel, "Kokainismus und Homosexualitat" (*Dtsch. Med. Wochenschr.* 51 (1925): 1562).

40. H. Piouffle, *Les Psychose Cocaïniques* (Paris: A. Maloine et fils, 1919).

41. N. Marx, "Beitrage zur Psychologie der Cocainomanie" (*Z. Ges. Neurol. Psychiat.* 80 (1922): 550).

42. H. Maier, *Der Kokainismus,* pp. 235–9.

43. *Ibid.,* pp. 246–8.

44. *Ibid.,* p. 240.

45. *Ibid.,* p. 241.

46. *Ibid.,* pp. 249–54.

47. V. Heinemann, *Medizinische und Psychologische Erfahrungen und Uberlegungen zur Schaffung einer Gesetzgebung gegen Kokain-Missbrauch* (Zurich: A. Oelschlager, 1923).

48. H. Zangger, "Diskussionsbermerkung zu dem Vortrag von Maier über Kokainismus" (*Schweiz. Arch. Neurol. Psychiatr.* 11 (1922): 144).

49. H. Maier, *Der Kokainismus,* pp. 253–63.

50. *Ibid.,* p. 59.

51. *Ibid.,* p. 261.

52. *Ibid.,* p. 262.

53. *Ibid.,* p. 263.

Chapter 10   Restrictive Laws against Cocaine: From National to International Legislation

1. David Musto, *The American Disease: Origins of Narcotic Control* (New York: Oxford University Press, 1987), pp. 8–10. This book is the most thoroughly documented text available on the history of drug addiction in the United States. It was extensively consulted in the writing of this chapter.

2. M. J. Wilbert and M. G. Motter, *Digest of Laws and Regulations in Force in the United States Relating to the Possession, Use, Sale and Manufacture of Poisons and Habit-Forming Drugs* (Washington, D.C.: U.S. Treasury Department, 1912).

3. Theodore Roosevelt (1858–1919). Twice President of the United States (1901–1909). Under his leadership the United States was established as a world power. In 1912 he became the standard-bearer of the Progressive movement, split the Republican party, and lost, to Woodrow Wilson, his third bid for the presidency of the United States.

4. In later years this Bureau was moved to the Department of Health. Dr. Wiley pioneered the fight against food additives and beverages containing not only "narcotic" drugs but also synthetic substances such as saccharin. The latter attempt irritated President Theodore Roosevelt, who consumed the sugar substitute daily. Wiley was forced out of government service in 1912 because of his uncompromising stand on the necessity of eliminating all potentially toxic substances from food and beverages.

5. Musto, p. 23.

6. *Ibid.*, pp. 23–4

7. *Ibid.*, pp. 25–8.

8. *Ibid.*

9. *Ibid.*, p. 27.

10. *Ibid.*, p. 28.

11. *Ibid.*, p. 30.

12. *Ibid.*, p. 31.

13. *Ibid.*, pp. 31, 38–40, 49–50, 61–2.

14. *Ibid.*, pp. 40–8.

15. *Ibid.*, pp. 49–53.

16. *Ibid.*, pp. 54–68.

17. Hamilton Wright estimated that there were 175,000 opium addicts in 1909, a figure close to the 200,000 reported by

the American Pharmaceutical Association in 1902. Adding to this figure 75,000 cocaine addicts, the figure of 250,000 seems a reasonable one. See Musto, p. 292, note 40.

18. Musto, pp. 56–8. Until 1914 the American Medical Association welcomed Federal government collaboration to achieve its professional goals.

19. *Ibid.,* pp. 56–8.

20. *Ibid.,* pp. 58, 83.

21. *Ibid.,* pp. 57–8.

22. National health insurance similar to that existing in all European countries has been opposed by the American Medical Association since the 1920s.

23. Musto, p. 297.

24. He was accused of drinking heavily (see Musto, p. 61). After his premature and accidental death in 1917 at the age of 49, his wife Elizabeth pursed his fight for strong antinarcotic legislation until her own death in 1952.

25. Dr. Jin Fuey Moy was a physician from Pittsburgh who had been indicted for prescribing opium to an opium addict. The district judge had quashed the indictment — a decision upheld by the U.S. Supreme Court in 1916. As a result of this decision, the Commissioner of the Treasury who administered the Harrison Act claimed that "it was practically impossible to control illicit traffic in narcotic drugs by unregistered persons" (Musto, pp. 128–31).

26. After the *Jin Fuey Moy* decision, amendments to the Harrison Act were requested from Congress in order to "facilitate restricting or eradicating entirely the use of narcotics for other than medicinal purposes," as stated in the 1916 report of the Commissioner of Internal Revenue. The 1919 decision of the Supreme Court, which reversed its 1916 decision, reflects a shift in thinking from concern for individual rights and quashing federal intervention to a belief that maintenance of addiction, even by medical prescription, represents an insuperable social danger (see Musto, pp. 327–8).

27. Musto, p. 145. DuMez' commentaries are complemented by those of Dr. Pearce Bailey, former chief neuropsychiatrist for the Army: "Drug addiction has too long been considered a medical problem. The problem is not one to be handled by the Board of Health, but by Internal Revenue Department to check up all sales, by municipal

police and by local and federal courts." (Musto, p. 333, note 68.)

28. Musto, pp. 134–82. Half of these clinics were located in New York state and New England. Others were located in the solid South: Shreveport, New Orleans, and Atlanta.

29. *Ibid.*, p. 149. There was little evidence that the maintenance clinics effected cures. Even the clinics that were well-run and had competent medical direction did not claim a large number of cures but, rather, "social adjustment" of the addicts.

30. *Ibid.*, p. 186. Dr. J. F. Rooney, an opponent of legislation that would restrain any of the prescription rights of physicians, was elected president of the New York State Medical Society in 1921.

31. *Ibid.*, p. 188. A three to six decision of the Court on 9 April 1928 (*Nigro v. U.S.*, 276 U.S. 332).

32. *Ibid.*, pp. 146–50 and 182–5.

33. *Ibid.*, p. 197. The Act was designed to limit exports to nations which had ratified the Hague Convention.

34. *Ibid.*, pp. 200–02. Porter hoped that passage of this bill would induce other nations to pass similar legislation, which, in effect, would ban manufacture of heroin all over the world.

35. *Ibid.*, pp. 202–04.

36. The Senate, which approved the participation of the American delegation to the Second Geneva Conference, stipulated that the U.S. would not sign an agreement which did not contain "the conditions necessary for the suppression of the habit forming narcotic traffic." See Musto, p. 202 and p. 355, note 66.

37. Musto, p. 203.

38. R. Giroux, "Etude clinique de l'intoxication par la cocaïne" (*Gaz. Hôp. Paris* 92 (1919): 245).

39. V. Cyril and Berger, *La "Coco," Poison Moderne* (Paris: Ernest Flammarion, 1924), and H. Maier, *Der Kokainismus,* p. 55.

40. H. Maier, *Der Kokainismus,* pp. 56–60.

41. Musto, pp. 214–16.

42. *Ibid.*, pp. 209–19. "The international aspects [of the narcotic problem]," said Porter, are "more important than the domestic," and the new Commissioner would need to be versed in "diplomatic wiles."

43. Musto, pp. 146-7.
44. *Annual Report[s] of the Commissioner of Prohibition,* 1927-1930. These figures have been disputed by Alfred Lindesmith in *The Addict and the Law* (Vintage Press, 1965, first published by Indiana University Press), pp. 104-22. His arguments are not convincing, and it appears that during the 1920s and 1930s, as a result of the vigorous interdiction measures applied by the Narcotics Division of the Prohibition Bureau and the Federal Bureau of Narcotics, there was a marked decline in addiction. This decline occurred within a cultural climate of social refusal of addictive drugs, widely supported by the media.
45. Musto, p. 204.
46. *Ibid.,* p. 205.
47. Daniel Price, Senate Subcommittee Hearings to Evaluate Narcotics Problems, June 2-8, 1955. Testimony of Harry Anslinger, pp. 9-10.
48. Musto, p. 214.
49. *Ibid.,* p. 234.
50. *Ibid.,* pp. 210-29. According to Anslinger, the pressure for Federal anti-marijuana laws had strong political support from local, state, and federal elected officials and statesmen (p. 223).
51. *Ibid.,* p. 220.
52. M. L. Harney and J. C. Cross, *The Narcotic Officer's Notebook* (Springfield, IL: Charles Thomas, 1965).
53. G. G. Nahas, "Hashish and Drug Abuse in Egypt during the 19th and 20th Centuries" (*Bulletin of the New York Academy of Medicine* 61 (1985): 428-44).
54. J. H. Anslinger and F. H. Tompkins, *The Traffic in Narcotics,* p. 265. During World War II, the rejection rate of draftees on the grounds of addiction was one in 10,000, compared to one in 1000 during World War I. And yet Lindesmith disputes these figures and claims that there was no decrease in the rate of addiction in the U.S. population between 1920 and 1942!
55. The Boggs Act passed on November 2, 1951. It was supported by Elizabeth Wright, the widow of Dr. Hamilton Wright.
56. Narcotic Control Act of 1956, Public Law 728, passed July 18, 1956.

57. N. Eddy, American physician and pharmacologist. He was Executive Secretary Commissioner on Drug Addiction and Narcotics, National Academy of Sciences, National Research Council (1961–1967) and consultant to the World Health Organization on addiction-producing drugs (1948–1965). Harry Isbell, professor of pharmacology, University of Kentucky Medical School, Lexington, Kentucky.

58. W.H.O. (World Health Organization) Technical Report Series 1952, no. 57, section 7, p. 11; and 1961, no. 211, section 3, p. 11.

Chapter 11   The Re-opening of Pandora's Box

1. Musto, p. 359, note 10.
2. *Ibid.,* note 11.
3. *Ibid.,* note 12.
4. To recognize his major contribution to the field of addiction, the faculty of the University of Indiana awarded Lindesmith the title of University Professor.
5. Lindesmith, The Addict and the Law. New York: Vintage Press, 1965, p. 170.
6. M. M. Glatt, "United Kingdom," pp. 145–70 in *The Community Response to Drug Use,* ed. S. Einstein (New York: Pergamon Press, 1980).
7. John Stuart Mill, "On Liberty," in *Philosophic Problems: An Introductory Book of Readings,* ed. M. Mandelbaum, F. W. Gramlich, and A. R. Anderson (New York: Macmillan, 1957).
8. Musto, p. 266.
9. *Ibid.,* pp. 234–5.
10. *Ibid.,* pp. 230–7.
11. *Ibid.,* p. 242.
12. Lindesmith, p. 96.
13. *Ibid.,* p. 238.
14. Musto, pp. 241–2.
15. *Ibid.,* p. 237.
16. Lindesmith, pp. 273–4.
17. G. G. Nahas, *Marijuana, Deceptive Weed* (New York: Raven Press, 1973), p. 75; and G. G. Nahas, *Keep Off the Grass* (Middlebury, VT: Eriksson, 1985), pp. 57–8.
18. *Ibid.,* pp. 201–02.

19. C. G. Nahas, *Marijuana: Deceptive Weed,* pp. 267–8.

20. S. Lesse, "Surprise, Doctor: Pot Is Here to Stay" (*American Journal of Psychotherapy* 25 (1971): 1–3).

21. E. Goode, *The Marijuana Smokers* (New York: Basic Books, 1970).

22. J. Kaplan, *Marijuana, the New Prohibition* (New York: World Press, 1971).

23. Grinspoon, *Marijuana Reconsidered.*

24. H. Brill, a psychiatrist and state official, specialized in the study of addictions. With Eddy and A. Wikler, he supported interdiction measures.

25. N. B. Eddy (1898–1975). American pharmacologist. He specialized in the study of narcotics and favored strong interdiction measures. He was executive secretary of the Committee on Drug Addiction and Narcotics of the National Academy of Sciences.

26. A. Wikler, American pharmacologist who studied the effects of narcotics in the Lexington federal facility for adults.

27. L. Grinspoon, review of *Marijuana: Deceptive Weed,* by C. G. Nahas, in the *New England Journal of Medicine* 288 (1973): 292–3; N. Zinberg, review of the same book in *Contemporary Drug Problems* (1973), pp. 341–5.

28. Report of the National Commission on Marijuana, "A Signal on Misunderstanding." See G. Nahas and A. Greenwood, *The First Report of the National Commission on Marijuana* (1972) and "Signal of Misunderstanding or Exercise in Ambiguity" *Bulletin of the New York Academy of Medicine,* 50 (1974): 55–75).

29. P. Anderson, *High in America: The True Story Behind NORML and the Politics of Marijuana* (New York: Viking Press, 1981). The book describes the rise and fall of Keith Stroup, the founder of the National Organization for the Reform of Marijuana Laws.

30. *Ibid.,* pp. 194–203; 308–13.

31. *Ibid.,* pp. 61, 95, 96.

32. *Ibid.,* 52–3, 66, 132, 218, 289, 308–09.

33. *Ibid.,* p. 218.

Chapter 12   The Cultural Acceptance of "Recreational" Drug Use in America

1. H. C. Frick, "A Study in Contrast: Books on Addictive Drugs printed in the U.S. (1970–1980)," in *Drug Abuse in the Modern World,* ed. G. G. Nahas and H. C. Frick (New York: Pergamon Press, 1981).

2. Brecher and the editors of *Consumers' Union, Licit and Illicit Drugs* (Boston: Little Brown and Co., 1972).

3. V. Rubin and L. Comitas, *Ganja in Jamaica* (The Hague: Mouton, 1975).

4. William Daniel Drake, Jr., *The Connoisseur Handbook of Marijuana* (San Francisco: Straight Arrow Books, 1971).

5. *The Gourmet Coke Book,* published anonymously (Calif.: White Mountain Press, Inc., 1972).

6. M. Lieberman, *The Dope Book* (New York: Praeger, 1978).

7. G. Rusoff, *The Gourmet Guide to Grass* (Los Angeles: Pinnacle Books, 1978).

8. Peter Stafford, *Psychedelic Baby Reaches Puberty* (New York: Dell, 1971).

9. R. C. Eng, *Responsible Drug and Alcohol Use* (New York: Macmillan, 1979).

10. W. Novak, *High Culture* (New York: Alfred A. Knopf, 1980).

11. V. Pawlak, *Drug Abuse: A Realistic Primer for Parents* (Phoenix, AZ: Do It Now Foundation, National Media Center).

12. STASH (Student Association for the Study of Hallucinogens, Inc.), Madison, WI 53703, are publishers of *The Journal of Psychedelic Drugs.*

13. "News of the Week in Review," *New York Times,* Sunday Ed., Aug. 1981.

14. William Burroughs, *Naked Lunch* (New York: Grove Press, 1959).

15. David Martin, "Marijuana and the Media," in Nahas and Frick, ed., *Drug Abuse,* pp. 164–73.

16. James L. Goddard, book review of Grinspoon's *Marijuana Reconsidered, New York Times,* 27 June 1971. Dr. Goddard was the U.S. Federal Drug Administration commissioner 1966–68.

17. Emile Durkheim, *Le Suicide: Etude de sociologie* (Paris: Librairie Alcan, 1867. It was republished in 1930 by Presses Universitaires de France (Paris).

18. J. Taqi, "Approbation of Drug Usage in Rock and Roll Music," in *Bulletin of Narcotics* 21 (4) (1969): 29–35).

19. Richard Ashley, *Cocaine, Its History, Uses, and Effects* (New York: Warner Books, 1975), pp. 133–5.

20. L. Grinspoon and Bakalar, "Drug Dependence: Non-Narcotic Agents," pp. 1621–22 in *Comprehensive Textbook of Psychiatry,* 3d ed., ed. H. I. Kaplan, A. M. Freedman, and B. G. Sadock (Baltimore, MD: Williams & Wilkins, 1980).

21. Jerry Hopkins in *Rolling Stone* 81: 29 April 1971.

22. In 1988 two researchers from Fairleigh University in New Jersey reported that mice exposed to discordant sounds present marked impairment of learning and memory and alterations in brain tissue. (G. M. Schreckenberg and H. H. Bird, "Neural Plasticity of Mus Musculus in Response to Disharmonic Sound," *Bulletin of the New Jersey Academy of Science* 32 (2) (Fall, 1987): 77–86.)

23. According to *Variety,* the trade publication of the entertainment world, *Easy Rider* grossed $16 million in the U.S. while *Lawrence of Arabia* grossed $15 million and *A Man For All Seasons* grossed $13 million.

Chapter 13   After Marijuana: Heroin and Cocaine

1. Musto, p. 234.

2. *Ibid.,* p. 261. This law established five schedules for drugs, depending on their potential for "abuse and dependency" and their medical use. Schedule I covers drugs of high dependency potential and no accepted medical use (heroin, LSD, and marijuana). Schedule II includes drugs with high dependency potential but accepted medical use (morphine) and cocaine. Schedule III includes amphetamines and barbiturates. Schedule IV includes meprobamate while Schedule V includes mixtures containing a low concentration of opiates, such as codeine. Penalties for dispensing illegally or for trafficking in any of these substances are related to their classification in these Schedules, the highest penalty being reserved for Schedule I drugs. No minimum penalty is defined. The penalty for first offense possession of small amounts of marijuana is probation for one year.

3. *Ibid.,* p. 263. NIDA was first headed by Dr. Robert Dupont, a psychiatrist who, after advocating the decriminalization of marijuana, courageously reversed his stand and lost his position.

4. *Ibid.*, p. 259.
5. V. P. Dole and M. E. Nyswander, "A Medical Treatment for Heroin Addiction" (*Journal of the American Medical Association* 193 (1965): 80).
6. For a review of methadone programs see Joyce H. Lowinson, "Methadone Maintenance in Perspective," pp. 344–54 in *Substance Abuse, Clinical Problems and Perspectives,* ed. Joyce H. Lowinson and Pedro Ruiz (Baltimore, MD: Williams and Wilkins, 1981).
7. See, for example, John N. Chappel, "Methadone and Chemotherapy in Drug Addiction—Genocidal or Lifesaving?" (*Journal of the American Medical Association* 228 (1974): 725–8).
8. Clonidine was introduced by Dr. M. Gold as a nonaddictive treatment of opiate addiction.
9. A. G. DuMez, "Some Facts Concerning Drug Addiction," a memorandum to the Surgeon General, 9 Dec. 1918, in Musto, p. 333, notes 65 and 68.
10. Anne Crittenden and Michael Ruby, "Cocaine, the Champagne of Drugs," *New York Times Magazine,* 1 Sept. 1974, p. 14.
11. Richard Woodley, *Dealer: Portrait of A Cocaine Merchant* (Warner paperback, 1972).
12. Bruce Jay Freiedman, *About Harry Towns* (New York: Alfred A. Knopf, 1974).
13. Richard Ashley, *Cocaine.*
14. *Ibid.*, p. 139.
15. *The Gourmet Coke Book.* See note 5, chapter 12.
16. W. Golden Mortimer, *Peru: History of Coca.* And/or Press Berkeley California 1974.
17. "Drugs and Drug Abuse" (*Education Newsletter* 3 (Aug. 1974): 5).
18. Lester Grinspoon and J. B. Bakalar, "Drug Dependence: Non–Narcotic Agents." See note 20, Chapter 12.
19. Lester Grinspoon and J. B. Bakalar, *Cocaine.* (New York: Basic Books, 1975). This volume includes an extensive bibliography.
20. Norman Zinberg is a professor of psychiatry at Harvard University. He is an advocate of responsible drug use and has written widely on this subject. See N. Zinberg and J. A. Robertson, *Drugs and the Public* (New York: Simon and Schuster, 1972).
21. Andrew Weil, a pupil of Norman Zinberg's, also advocates

"recreational use" of addictive drugs. He is a prolific author on this subject. See note 3, Chapter 22.

22. R. Clayton and H. Voss, *U. S. Journal of Drug and Alcohol Dependence,* Jan. 1982.

23. D. Kandel, "Stages in Adolescent Involvement in Drug Use" (*Science* 190 (1975): 912).

24. "Drug Abuse," a Domestic Council Drug Review task force white paper for the President (Washington, D.C.: U.S. Government Printing Office, 1975), pp. 37–9.

25. C. V. Wetli and R. K. Wright, "Death Caused by Recreational Cocaine Use" (*Journal of the American Medical Association* 241 (1979): 1519–22.

Chapter 14   Cocaine, the Intellectual Establishment, and the Parents of America

1. *Facts About Drug Abuse* by the Drug Abuse Council (New York: The Free Press, a division of Macmillan, 1980, p. iv), hereafter referred to as *Facts About Drug Abuse.* The book has a foreword by M. Webster Bethuel, the chairman of the Drug Abuse Council.

2. Lindesmith, *Addict and the Law.*

3. *Facts About Drug Abuse,* p. iv.

4. *Drug Abuse Council I.R.S. Tax Returns* (New York: The Foundation Center, 1971, 1972, 1974–78).

5. *Facts About Drug Abuse,* pp. vi–vii.

6. Anderson, *High in America,* p. 98.

7. *Facts About Drug Abuse,* p. 19.

8. "A First Report of the Impact of California's New Marijuana Laws (SB 95)" (California Health and Welfare Agency, State Office of Narcotics and Drug Abuse, January 1977), pp. 7–8.

9. S. Rusche, "The Drug Abuse Council," pp. 205–12 in *Drug Abuse in the Modern World* (New York: Pergamon Press, 1981).

10. L. D. Johnston, J. C. Bachman, and P. M. O'Malley, *Drug Use Among American High School Students* (Rockville, MD: National Institute on Drug Abuse, 1975–1979). This work is published annually.

11. *Facts About Drug Abuse,* p. 188.

12. *Ibid.,* pp. 185–7.

13. *Ibid.,* p. 4.

14. A. Weil and W. Rosen, *Chocolate to Morphine: Understanding Mind-Active Drugs* (Boston: Houghton Mifflin, 1983). This book was recommended reading to teenagers in the popular column, "Ask Beth," published in *The Boston Globe Magazine,* Sunday ed., 24 February 1985.

15. *Ibid.,* "Straight Talk at the Start," p. 1.

16. *Ibid.,* p. 3.

17. *Ibid.*

18. *Ibid.,* p. 86. Weil classifies opiates among the depressants, along with minor tranquilizers, barbiturates, and general anesthetics.

19. *Ibid.,* p. 85. A most erroneous claim. Opiates are known to attach to receptors of the lymphocytes, the main cells of the immunity system. As a result, the opiate addict has a lowered resistance to infection.

20. *Ibid.,* p. 120.

21. *Ibid.,* p. 47.

22. *Ibid.,* p. 56.

23. Shervert Frazier, professor of psychiatry at Harvard University, and Daniel X. Freedman, professor of psychiatry at the University of Chicago, had a great influence on appointments to NIDA, NIMH,. and ADAMHA.

24. *Facts About Drug Abuse,* p. 57, and *FASEB Bulletin,* July 1987.

25. Robert Byck, M.D., a member of the department of psychiatry at Yale University. He was the recipient of NIDA grant 5R01DA-01873 for fiscal years 1977–79 in the amount of $426,237 to study "cocaine effects and modification of euphoria in man."

26. Peggy Mann, *Marijuana Alert* (New York: Macmillan, 1984).

27. Nahas, *Keep Off the Grass* (Middlebury, VT: Eriksson, 1984). This book gives some examples of NIDA's cautious approach.

28. "Research Issues #8, A Cocaine Bibliography Non-Annotated" (NIDA, December 1974), p. 56.

29. "Research Issues #15." Cocaine summaries of psychosocial research (NIDA, 1975).

30. *NIDA Research Monograph 13, Cocaine 1977,* ed. R. C. Petersen and R. C. Stillman (Rockville, MD: NIDA, 1977).

31. *Ibid.*, R. L. Dupont, foreword, pp. v–vi.

32. *Ibid.*, pp. 1–4.

33. R. Byck and C. Van Dyke, "What are the Effects of Cocaine on Man?" (*Nida Research Monograph 13*, pp. 97–114).

34. The sum allotted by NIDA to Robert Byck, the principal investigator, from fiscal year 1974 through fiscal year 1980 was $1,054,936. This was for two grants, which sometimes ran concurrently (R01DA–0057) and (ADM–45–74–164).

35. R. K. Siegel, "Cocaine: Recreational Use and Intoxication" (*NIDA Research Monograph 13* (1977), pp. 119–36).

36. D. Briand, "Un Singe Cocaïnomane 'Bullet' " (*Soc. Clin. Med. Ment.* 16 (1913), p. 182).

37. D. R. Wesson and D. E. Smith, "Cocaine: Its Use for Central Nervous System Stimulation Including Recreational and Medical Use" (*NIDA Research Monograph 13*, pp. 137–52).

38. B. S. Finkle and K. L. McCloskey, "The Forensic Toxicology of Cocaine" (*NIDA Research Monograph 13*, pp. 152–92).

39. G. G. Nahas, *Marijuana in Science and Medicine* (New York: Raven Press, 1985).

40. All grants awarded by NIDA undergo a careful review by committees of scientific peers. But it seems that some committees have much larger funds at their disposal than others. Furthermore, some investigators seem to be more readily selected by their peers.

41. American Council for Drug Education, 5820 Hubbard Drive, Rockville, MD 20857.

42. PRIDE (Parents Resource Institute for Drug Education), The Hurt Building, 50 Hurt Plaza, Atlanta, GA 30303.

43. National Federation of Parents for a Drug Free Youth (N.F.P.), Washington, D.C.

44. Committees of Correspondence, Inc., Drug Awareness Information, 57 Conant St., Danvers, MA 01923 (phone 617-774-2641).

45. S. Cohen, *Cocaine Today* (Rockville, MD: American Council for Drug Education, 1982).

Chapter 15   From Icy Norway to California Snow, 1982

1. Eric Clapton, "Cocaine," lyrics by J. J. Cale, 1975.

2. Nicholas Von Hoffman, "The Cocaine Culture, New

Wave for the High and Hip," *Washington Post,* 23 April 1975.

3. M. M. McCarron and J. D. Wood, "The Cocaine Body Packer Syndrome" (*Journal of the American Medical Association* 250 (1984): 1417–20).

4. Report of Seizures, Drug Enforcement Agency, 1982.

5. New York State Department of Public Health, Controlled Substances Division, 1975 to 1981 *Reports.*

6. L. D. Johnston, J. G. Bachman, and P. M. O'Malley, *Student Drug Use in America* (University of Michigan Institute for Social Research); "Trends in Prevalence 1980–82" (Rockville, MD: NIDA, Division of Research, 1983).

7. E. H. Adams and J. Durrell, "Cocaine: A Growing Public Health Problem" and "Cocaine: Pharmacology, Effects of Abuse" (*NIDA Research Monograph #50* (1984), pp. 9–14).

8. F. R. Jeri, C. C. Sanchez, T. del Pozo, M. Fernandez, and C. Carbajal, "Further Experience with the Syndromes Produced by Coca Paste Smoking" (*Narcotics Bulletin* 30 (3) (1978): 1–11).

9. W. Pollin, foreword to *Cocaine: Pharmacology, Effects and Treatment of Abuse,* ed. J. Grabowski (*NIDA Research Monograph #50* (1984), p. vii.

10. *Ibid.,* p. viii.

11. R. T. Jones, "The Pharmacology of Cocaine," in *Cocaine: Pharmacology, Effects and Treatment of Abuse* (*NIDA Research Monograph #50* (1984), p. 46).

12. R. K. Siegel, "Changing Patterns of Cocaine Use: Longitudinal Observations, Consequences, and Treatment," in *Cocaine: Pharmacology, Effects and Treatment of Abuse,* ed. J. Grabowski (*NIDA Research Monograph #50* (1984), pp. 92–110).

13. H. D. Kleber and F. H. Gawin, "Cocaine Abuse: A Review of Current and Experimental Treatments," in *Cocaine: Pharmacology, Effects and Treatment of Abuse (NIDA Research Monograph #50* (1984), pp. 111–29).

Chapter 16   An Academic Confrontation on Cocaine

1. Sidney Cohen, M.D., Ph.D., professor of psychiatry at the University of California at Los Angeles.

2. Siegel, "Changing Patterns." The presentation given by Dr. Siegel in Santa Monica was similar to that delivered at the NIDA conference of 1982, described in the previous chapter.
3. Nahas, "Pharmacological Classification," pp. 1–14. The classification is described in the table on pp. 276-277.
4. *Cocaine 1980: Proceedings of the Interamerican Seminar on Medical and Sociological Aspects of Coca and Cocaine* ed. F. R. Jeri (Lima, Peru: Pacific Press, 1980). These Proceedings are hereafter referred to as *Cocaine 1980*.
5. D. R. Wesson and D. E. Smith, "Cocaine: Treatment Perspectives," in *Cocaine Use in America: Epidemiologic and Clinical Perspectives,* ed. N. J. Kozel and E. H. Adams (*NIDA Research Monograph #61* (1985), pp. 193–203).

Chapter 17   Dr. Timothy Leary and the Media

1. Dr. Timothy Leary described his experiences in his books *The Policy of Ecstasy* (New York: Putnam, 1968) and *Flashbacks* (Calif.: J. P. Tarcher, Inc., 1985).
2. Aldous Huxley, *The Doors of Perception* (New York: Harper Bros., 1954).
3. Albert Hofmann, world-renowned organic chemist, head of the Pharmaceutical Chemical Research Laboratories of Sandoz Laboratories in Basel, Switzerland. Before World War II he synthesized lysergic acid diethylamide (L.S.D.). It is a derivative from ergot, a fungus which is a parasite of rye. In 1943 Hofmann accidentally discovered the hallucinogenic effects of LSD. Deeply impressed by the effects of minute amounts on his perception of the universe, Hofmann went on to experiment with the drug. He gave an account of his experience in his book, *LSD: My Problem Child* (translated by Jonathan Ott (Los Angeles: J. P. Tarcher, Inc., 1983, distributed by Houghton Mifflin [Boston])). Hofmann genuinely believed that LSD, when carefully used under medical supervision, could be a useful drug for the "self exploration" of the unconscious. He confirmed his experiences with Aldous Huxley and the novelist Ernst Junger. Widespread experimentation with LSD in the 1950s, by people less reasonable and with more vulnerable brains than those of Huxley and Hofmann, led to bad trips, panic, flashbacks, depression, paranoia, psychotic episodes, and suicide. In 1965 Sandoz Laboratories stopped fabricating and distribut-

ing LSD. The drug was banned from public consumption in the U.S. and placed on Schedule I (dangerous drugs with no medical application), along with heroin.

4. Psilocybin, an hallucinogenic substance, is the active ingredient of a Mexican mushroom, Psilocybe Mexicana. It was also synthesized by Hofmann.

Chapter 18   Cousteau's Explorers Discover Cocaine in the Amazon Jungle

1. The seven TV films of Cousteau's Amazon expedition have been projected all over the world. They may be obtained in video cassettes from The Cousteau Society, 425 E. 52nd St., New York, NY 10022 (telephone 212-826-2940). The "Calypso" is the ship from which Cousteau has led his expeditions throughout the oceans and water–ways of the world for over three decades.

2. *"Front Populaire sur l'altiplano: La Coca, un Etat dans l'Etat," Le Monde,* 23 April 1983.

3. Nahas, *Keep Off the Grass,* 4th ed., with a preface by Jacques Yves Cousteau (Middlebury, VT: Eriksson, 1984).

4. Luis Martin, *The Kingdoms of the Sun: A Short History of Peru* (New York: Charles Scribners and Son, 1974).

Chapter 19   When Cocaine Becomes the Religion of a People

1. D. Paly, P. Jatlow, C. Van Dyke, F. Cabieses, and R. Byck, "Plasma Levels of Cocaine in Native Peruvian Coca Chewers," in *Cocaine 1980,* pp. 86–9.

2. W. E. Carter, P. Parkerson, and M. Mamani, "Traditional and Changing Patterns of Coca Use in Bolivia," in *Cocaine 1980,* pp. 159–64.

3. Phenothiazine, a major tranquilizer used in the treatment of schizophrenia and of acute psychosis.

4. Carlos Noriega Gutierrez and Vicente Zapata Ortiz, *Estudios sobre la Coca y la Cocaina en el Peru* (Lima, Peru: Lima Ministerio de Educacion Publica, 1947).

5. D. Paly, et al., *Cocaine 1980,* pp. 86–9.

6. In spite of successive land and social reforms, Peru's population is still divided between the "haves" and "have nots," with a small middle class and a very large number of destitute

Common Properties of Addictive Drugs
(from Nahas, *Keep Off the Grass*, Eriksson, 1984)

Drugs	1 Pleasure Reward	2 Neuropsychological impairment (reversible)	3 Withdrawal symptoms	4 Tolerance	5 Reinforcement
Opiates					
Morphine	+	+++	+++	+++	+++
Heroin	+	+++	+++	+++	+++
Methadone	+	+	+	+	+
Synthetic agonists	+	+	+	+	+
Major Psychostimulants					
Cocaine	+	++	++	++	++
Amphetamine	+	++	++	++	++
Psychodepressants					
Alcohol*	+	+++	+++	+++	+++
Barbiturates	+	+++	+++	+++	+++
Benzodiazepines	+	+	+	+	+
Methaqualone	+	+	+	+	+
Cannabis					
Hashish	+	++	++	++	++
Marijuana, THC	+	++	++	++	++

Hallucinogens**					
LSD	+	+	0	+	+
Psilocybine	+	+	0	+	+
Mescaline	+	+	0	+	+
Anticholinergic (Datura, Belladona)	+	+	0	+	+
Phencyclidine (PCP)	+	+	0	+	+
Solvents					
Benzene, Toluene	+	+	0	+	+
Acetone	+	+	0	+	+
Trichloroethylene	+	+	0	+	+
Ether, N_2O, $CHCl_3$	+	+	0	+	+
Minor Psychostimulants					
Tobacco (Nicotine)***	+	0	+	+	+
Cola	+	0	+	+	+
Khat	+	0	+	+	+
Caffeine***	+	0	+	+	+

*Alcohol in small amounts does not induce psychological or physical impairment.
**Hallucinogens may induce severe mental reactions/"bad trips."
***Tobacco and caffeine do not produce neuropsycho-toxicity.

farmers, workers, and unemployed. The Communist revolution still holds a strong appeal among the masses.

Chapter 20   Treating the Pastaleros with Astronauts' Vitamins

1. Thorazine is the trade name for chlorpromazine, a major tranquilizer which revolutionized the treatment of schizophrenia and effectively restored these severely ill patients to coherently functioning individuals. Haldol (generic name butyrophenone) is another effective medication in the treatment of schizophrenia.

Chapter 21   Cocaine Addiction and Psychosurgery

1. Alcoholic polyneuritis is a painful inflammation of the nerves to the limbs. It is observed in chronic alcoholism and results from nutritional and vitamin B deficiency.
2. G. Burkhardt, Swiss surgeon and anatomist. He was the first to perform psychosurgery on a demented patient, as described in "Uber Rindenexcisionen, als Beitrag zur operativen Therapy der Psychosen" (*Allg. Ztschr. f. Psychiat.* 74 (1890): 463.
3. Antonia De Egas Moniz (1874–1955). Portuguese physician. Co-recipient, with W. R. Hess, of the Nobel Prize in medicine, for the discovery of the therapeutic value of prefrontal leucotomy in certain psychoses. Leucotomy is described in Moniz, *Tentatives Operatoires dans la Traîtment de Certaines Psychoses* 21 (Paris: Masson et Cie., 1936).
4. Prefrontal leucotomy is the surgical section of nerve bundles connecting the limbic area of the old brain to the frontal lobes. This was a blind procedure.
5. J. Le Beau, French neurosurgeon who perfected, in the early 1950s, the open cyngulotomy performed by the Peruvian surgeon on irretrievable cocaine addicts. He described his studies in the following papers: "Cingular and Precingular Areas in Psychosurgery (Agitated Behavior, Obsessive Compulsive States, Epilepsy)" (*Acta Psych. Neurol. Scand.*, 27 (1952): 304–16); "Comparison of Personality Changes After (1) Prefrontal Selective Surgery for the Re-

lief of Intractable Pain and for the Treatment of Mental Cases" and (2) "Cingulectomy and Topectomy" (*J. Ment. Sci.* 99 (1953): 53–61); "Anterior Cingulectomy in Man" (*J. Neurosurg.* 11: (1954): 268); and *Psycho-chirurgie et Fonctions Mentales: Techniques, Résultats, Applications Physiologiques* (Paris: Masson, 1954).

6. In India cyngulotomy was performed in the treatment of drug addiction by V. Balasubramanian, who described it in his work in "Surgery for Drug Addiction" (*Syringe* 1 (1971): 155–6); "Stereotaxic Cingulotomy for Drug Addiction" (*Neurology India* 21 (1973): 63); and "The Practice of Psychosurgery: A Survey of the Literature (1971–1976)" (cited in J. S. Stevens, *Psychosurgery,* U. S. Department of Health (OS) 77-0002, 1977, in the Appendix at p. 1).

7. Le Beau. See note 5, this chapter, and Le Beau's work referenced therein.

8. D. Kelly, "Stereotactic Limbic Leucotomy: Clinical, Psychological and Physiological Assessment at 16 Months," in W. H. Sweet, et al. (eds), *Neurosurgical Treatment in Psychiatry: Pain and Epilepsy* (Baltimore, MD: University Park Press, 1977).

9. K. E. Livingston, "Cingulate Cortex Isolation for the Treatment of Psychoses and Psychoneuroses" (*Ass. Res. Nerv. Ment. Dis. Proceedings* 31 (1951): 374); G. Rylander, "The Renaissance of Psychosurgery," in E. Hitchcock, et al. (eds.), *Psychosurgery* (Springfield, IL: Charles C. Thomas, 1972); H. T. Ballantine, "Frontal Cingulotomy for Mood Disturbance," p. 221 in Hitchcock; Ballantine, "Cingulotomy for Psychiatric Illness: Report of 13 Years' Experience," p. 333 in W. H. Sweet, et al., *Neurosurgical Treatment;* and S. Corkin, "Safety and Efficacy of Cingulotomy in Man for Pain or Psychiatric Disorders," p. 253 in E. R. Hitchcock, H. T. Ballantine, and B. A. Myerson (eds.), *Modern Concepts in Psychiatric Surgery* (Amsterdam: Elsevier-North Holland Publishing Co., 1979).

10. J. Gaches, "Sur L'action de la Topectomie dan les Douleurs Irréductibles: à propos de Deux Cas de Causalgie" (*Semaine d. Hôp. Paris* 2225 (1949): 2226).

11. V. Balasubramanian. See note 6, this chapter, and the works referenced therein.

12. Theobaldo Llosa. Follow-up study of twenty-eight coca

paste addicts treated by open cyngulotemy. VIIth World Congress of Psychiatry, Vienna, 1983.

13. Pierre Paul Broca (1824–1880). French surgeon, anatomist, and anthropologist. He investigated topography of the skull and brain and prehistoric trepanation of Peruvian skulls, which he described in "Cas Singulier de Trépanation chez les Incas" (Bull. Anthrop. Soc. Paris, 2e série, vol. 2, 1967), pp. 293–319.

14. J. H. Breasted, The Edwin Smith Surgical Papyrus (Chicago: University of Chicago Press, 1930). Also see C. A. Elsberg, "The Anatomy and Surgery of the Edwin Smith Papyrus" (J. Mt. Sinai Hosp. 12 (1945): 141–51).

15. Alex Hrdlicka, "Trepanation Among Prehistoric People, Especially in America" (Ciba Symposia, vol. 1 (1933), pp. 170–7).

16. Theobaldo Llosa's address is International Institute of Information on Coca and Derivatives, Los Olivos 364, San Isidro, Lima, Peru (telephone 22–2935).

Chapter 22   Tingo Maria: The White City

1. The high plateau of the Andes where the native Indian coca chewers, or coqueros, live and work as farmers and miners.

2. E.N.A.C.O. (Empressa Nacional de la Coca) is the Peruvian state monopoly which controls the area of licit cultivation of the coca bush. This licit cultivation is required to supply coca leaves to the Indians and the raw material for licit production of cocaine for medical uses.

3. A. T. Weil, "The Therapeutic Value of Coca in Contemporary Medicine" (Journal of Ethnopharmacology 3 (1981): 367–76). "Letters from Andrew Weil" (Journal of Psychedelic Drugs 7 (4) (1975): 401–13) and "Why Coca Leaf Should Be Available as a Recreational Drug" (Journal of Psychedelic Drugs 9 (1) (1977): 75–78) are two publications in which Weil has recommended that the natural extracts of the coca leaf be used for recreational purposes. Other books by this author include Chocolate to Morphine, with W. Rosen; The Marriage of the Sun and Moon: A Quest for Unity in Consciousness (Boston: Houghton Mifflin Co., 1980); and The Natural Mind: A New Way of Looking at Drugs and the Higher Consciousness (Boston: Houghton Mifflin Co., 1972).

Chapter 23   The Traffickers of Juan Juy

1. The guerrillas of the "Senderoso luminoso" (Shining Path) are fanatic revolutionaries akin to the bloody Cambodian partisans of Pol Pot. They have been fighting the government forces since the late seventies. Many of the thousands of victims have been the poor villagers caught in the cross fire.

Chapter 24   Consuming and Producing Countries: Shared Responsibilities

1. Beneficial Plant Research Association (1982), Carmel Valley, CA 93024. This non-profit scientific and educational corporation was formed in 1979 "to investigate and promote the use of plants to improve human life." Its main goal is to "preserve the natural composition of beneficial plants," by investigating methods of preparing plants to facilitate their distribution and use without isolating particular elements from them or refining them into unnatural forms.

   All of these claims are applied by the Beneficial Plant Research Association to the coca leaf, and the "coca project" is the first major undertaking of this humanitarian group. Indeed, their "field work and preliminary studies" have convinced them that "coca in natural form has great potential as a safe and effective therapeutic agent in modern medicine." It is their intent to manufacture a whole alcohol extract of the natural coca leaf containing all of the nutrients, essential oils, and alkaloids of the plant, including cocaine. Such a standardized solid or semi-solid whole extract of coca "can be processed into various forms, such as lozenges or chewing gum in which the contents of alkaloids would be the same as in the leaves." The extract would be made available to researchers and tested in animal and man for possible uses as a medicinal preparation in a host of conditions from digestive disturbances to obesity, which were reviewed a hundred years ago by Freud. The general claim is that, in natural form, coca is nontoxic and has a low potential for abuse.

   Other stimulants which are "safely effective and useful" will also be made available by the Beneficial Plant

Association, such as Khat (catha edulis), the traditional masticatory of Ethiopia and Yemen, whose leaf contains amphetamine-like compounds. Natural sedatives such as "Kava" will be investigated as alternative to the minor tranquilizers. The Association will also consider ways to educate people about the intelligent use of plants which affect mood, such as coca, khat, and kava. Indeed, the Association's contention is that "if employed carefully, these substances can be valuable medicine without harmful side effects," and that they can be used in a healthy fashion.

The goals of the Beneficial Plant Association are most laudable, but they are based on assumptions which empirical observation as well as scientific research have proved to be erroneous, especially when applied to stimulant substances. Indeed, man has always extracted from medicinal plants the biologically active molecules they contain, because they are easier to standardize, to store and transport, and to apply for their specific pharmacological properties.

When it comes to plants which contain substances having an abuse potential, such as cocaine, the desire and power of man to extract the psychoactive ingredient of the plant is considerably reinforced. Cocaine, which is contained in the coca leaf, affords the best example of the natural propensity of man to use and abuse any medicine containing this alkaloid. One century of observations have proven that cocaine is one of the most addictive drugs. Modern man, unlike the Andean miner, is able to consume the drug in a rapid, effortless fashion associated with euphoria. The W.H.O. committee on addictive drugs has concluded that cocaine is the *prototype* of stimulant drugs capable of inducing euphoric excitement.

2. A. A. Buck, T. T. Sasaki, J. J. Hewitt, and A. A. Macrae, "Coca Chewing and Health: An Epidemiologic Study Among Residents of a Peruvian Village" (*American Journal of Epidemiology* 88 (2) (1968): 159–77). A summary of this paper appears in *Bulletin of Narcotics* 22 (4) (1970): 23–32.

3. J. C. Negrete and H. B. M. Murphy, "Psychological Deficit in Chewers of Coca Leaf" (*Bulletin of Narcotics* 19 (4) (1967): 11–18).

4. Carter, Parkerson, and Mamani, in *Cocaine 1980*, pp. 159–64.

5. *Ibid.*, p. 162.

Chapter 25   The Cold War and the Business of Cocaine

1. Jacques Yves Cousteau and Jean–Michel Cousteau, *Snowstorm in the Jungle* (New York: Cousteau Society, 1984).
2. Nicollo Machiavelli (1469–1527). Italian statesman and writer, inventor of the reason of state which supersedes all others including moral commitments. His main books are *The Prince* and *The Discourses.*
3. U. S. Senate Committee on Internal Security Hearings, Sen. Paula Hawkins, chairman (Washington, D.C.: U. S. Government Printing Office, 1983).
4. P. Eddy, H. Sabogal, and S. Walden, *The Cocaine Wars* (New York: W. W. Norton, 1988).
5. *Ibid.,* pp. 141–7; 155–7.
6. *Ibid.,* pp. 334–8.
7. *Ibid.,* pp. 337–43.
8. Eddy, et al., *Cocaine Wars.*
9. M. Gold, *Cocaine 800* (New York: Bantam Books, 1984).
10. Afghanistan, Pakistan, and Iran constitute the "golden crescent" which now produces more heroin than the "golden triangle" of Burma, Thailand, and Laos.
11. G. G. Nahas, AMPART Report of U.S.I.A. on Visit to Warsaw, 28–30 November 1988.
12. Lidell Hart, *Strategy* (A Signet Book, New American Library, 1974).
13. *New York Times,* 20 April 1989, p. 24.
14. According to Dr. Miguel Solan Soteras, one of the officials responsible for the Spanish drug control program, Spain is in the process of becoming the main staging area for the traffic of cocaine into Europe. Several tons were seized in 1988; shipments of the order of 50 tons are expected in 1989. The frequent daily air and sea communications between Spain and South American Spanish-speaking countries account for the rapid development of the cocaine trade in Spain and make it difficult to control. With the elimination of customs barriers along the borders of the countries of the European community in 1992, a marked increase of cocaine traffic is expected in these countries. Alan Riding in *The New York Times,* 29 April 1989.

Chapter 26   The Experimental Administration of Cocaine to the Human and Nonhuman Primate

284   Gabriel G. Nahas

1. Musto, pp. 23–8. Under the leadership of President Theodore Roosevelt and Secretary of State John Hays, supported by Dr. Hamilton Wright, in 1908 the State Department became the leading proponent of national and international legislation to control addictive drugs.
2. In the past twenty years I have visited or lectured in Canada, Jamaica, the Bahamas, Brazil, Peru, Colombia, Venezuela, France, Belgium, Holland, Germany, England, Switzerland, Italy, Spain, Yugoslavia, Greece, Poland, Sweden, Norway, Finland, Egypt, Lebanon, Morocco, Kuwait, Singapore, Tahiti, and Australia.
3. Albert Camus, *The Plague* (New York: Alfred A. Knopf, 1948).
4. See Chapter 21, "Cocaine Addiction and Psychosurgery."
5. "Guidelines for Use of Experimental Animals" (National Institutes of Health, 1985).
6. The Addiction Research Center is directed by Dr. Jerome Jaffe, the first Director of Drug Abuse Policy of the White House, appointed by President Richard Nixon in 1974.
7. G. G. Nahas, R. Trouvé, W. M. Manger, C. Vinyard, and S. Goldberg, "Cocaine Cardiac Toxicity and Endogenous Catecholamines," in *Progress in Catecholamine Research,* ed. M. Sandler, A. Dahlstron, and R. H. Belmaker, (New York: Alan Liss, 1988), Part B, pp. 457–62.
8. G. G. Nahas, R. Trouvé, J. F. Demus, and M. Sitbon, "A Calcium Channel Blocker As an Antidote to the Cardiac Effects of Cocaine Intoxication" (*New England Journal of Medicine* 313 (1985): 8, p. 519 (correspondence)).
9. Marian W. Fischman and Charles R. Schuster, "Cocaine Self-Administration in Humans" (*Fed. Proc.* 41 (2) (1982): 241–46).
10. These studies of cocaine administration to cocaine addicts have been funded by the National Institute on Drug Abuse in the following institutions: Yale University, Department of Psychiatry, Dr. Robert Byck (from 1974–1980, funding of $1,054,436); University of Chicago, Department of Psychiatry, Dr. Charles R. Schuster and Dr. Marian Fischman (from 1977–1984, funding of $1,555,980); University of California at San Francisco, Dr. Reese Jones (from 1981–1985, funding of $340,077). This list is not exhaustive. Other studies have also been performed since 1966 at Johns Hopkins University, Department of Psychiatry (Dr.

Marian Fischman); Northwestern University, Department of Clinical Pharmacology (Dr. John J. Ambre); and the Addiction Research Center, Baltimore, Maryland (Dr. Jerome Jaffe).

11. Dr. Jerome Jaffe.

12. Dr. Charles R. Schuster.

13. NIDA Science Policy Subcommittee, Dr. Charles O'Brien, chairman, 4 May 1987. Topic: Experimental use of cocaine in human subjects.

14. "Scientific Perspectives on Cocaine Abuse," American Society for Pharmacology and Experimental Therapeutics and Committee on Problems of Drug Dependence (*The Pharmacologist* 29 (1987): 20–7).

15. R. T. Jones, "Clinical and Behavioral Considerations in Emission Tomography Study Design," in *NIDA Research Monograph 74, Neurobiology of Behavioral Control in Drug Abuse* (1986), pp. 117–23.

16. All of these references are given in a paper by G. G. Nahas, "The Experimental Use of Cocaine in Man: A Point of View" (*Bulletin of Narcotics* (1989)).

17. H. D. Tazelaar, S. B. Karch, B. G. Stephens, and M. E. Billingham, "Cocaine and the Heart" (*Human Pathology* 18 (1987): 195–9).

18. See Nahas, Trouvé, Manger, Vinyard and Goldberg, "Cocaine Cardiac Toxicity," and Nahas, Trouvé, Demus, and Sitbon, "Calcium Channel Blocker." See also G. G. Nahas, R. Trouvé, and M. Maillet, "Prevention of the Cardiotoxicity of Cocaine by Nitrendipine, a Ca2 + Blocker" (*Bulletin Académie Nationale Médécine* 169 (1985): 1151–6), and R. Trouvé and G. Nahas, "Nitrendipine: An Antidote to Cardiac and Lethal Toxicity of Cocaine" (*Proc. Soc. Exptl. Biol. Med.* 183 (1986): 392–7).

19. L. Shuster and M. L. Thompson, "Epinephrine and Liver Damage from Cocaine" (*The Pharmacologist* 27 (1985): 200); L. Shuster, F. Quimby, A. Bates, and M. L. Thompson, "Liver Damage from Cocaine in Mice" (*Life Sci.* 20 (1977): 1035–42); E. Bravetta and G. Invernizzi, "Il Cocainismo: Osservazione Cliniche Ricerche Sperimentali e Anatomopatologiche" (*Note Riv. Psichiatr.* 10 (1922): 543; 11 (1923): 179).

20. Tazelaar, Karch, Stephens, and Billingham.

21. Harrison Act of 1914 (Musto, pp. 59–61, 62–5).

22. In 1919 and again in 1928 the U.S. Supreme Court ruled that maintenance of addiction, even by medical prescription, represents an insuperable social danger which overrides concern for individual rights (Musto, pp. 128-30, 185, 187). The cases are *U.S. v. Doremus*, 249 U.S. 86 (March 3, 1919), and *Nigro v. U.S.*, 276 U.S. 332 (April 9, 1928).
23. Helsinki Declaration on Human Rights, 1977.

Chapter 27   Cocaine Addiction, A Self-Inflicted Impairment of Brain Neurotransmission

1. R. Heath, *The Role of Pleasure in Behavior* (New York: Hoeber Medical Division, Harper and Row, 1964).
2. Blaise Pascal (1623-1662). French mathematician, physician, and natural philosopher. This quotation is from his *Pensees*.
3. It is on this hypothesis that the cyngulotomy operation has been performed in Peru to relieve the compulsion of cocaine addiction.
4. This hypothesis is discussed in G. Nahas and R. Trouve: Dépendance à la cocaine et perturbation de la neurotransmission cèrébrale Bull. Acad. Notle. Med. 173 (1989).
5. Nahas, R. Trouvé, and Maillet, "Prevention of Cardiotoxicity," pp. 392-7; R. Trouvé and G. Nahas, "Nitrendipine: An Antidote to Cardiac and Lethal Toxicity of Cocaine" (*Proc. Soc. Exptl. Biol. Med.* 183 (1986): 392-7); R. Trouvé and G. Nahas, "Interactions de la Cocaine et de l'angiotensine" (*Bull. Acad. Natle. Med.* 172 (1988): 841-845).
6. L. Cote and L. T. Kremzner, "Biochemical Changes in Normal Aging in the Human Brain," pp. 19-30 in *The Dementias*, ed. R. Mayeux and W. G. Rosen (New York: Raven Press, 1983).
7. Arthur Koestler, *Janus, A Summing Up* (New York: Hutchinson, 1979).
8. Claude Bernard (1813-1878). French physician and founder of modern physiology. His book, *Introduction à la Médecine Expérimentale*, formulated the main rules of biological experimentation. He held that body mechanisms strive to maintain a constant inner environment through feedback regulations.

9. Walter Bradley Cannon (1871–1945). American physiologist, author of *The Wisdom of the Body* (1932) in which he defines "homeostasis."

10. Marcel Proust, *Remembrance of Things Past* (New York: Modern Library, 1929).

11. J. S. Mill, "On Liberty."

12. Charles Baudelaire, *Les Paradis Artificiels* (Paris: Livre de Poche, 1972).

13. J. J. Moreau, *Du Hashish et de L'aliénation Mentale* (Paris: Masson, 1846). There is an English translation, *Hashish and Mental Illness*, edited by H. Peters and G. Nahas (New York: Raven Press, 1983).

Chapter 28   The Epidemic Spread of Cocaine and Its
           Containment

1. N. Bejerot, *Addiction and Society* (Springfield, IL: Charles C. Thomas, 1970). By the same author: *Addiction, an Artificially-induced Drive* (Springfield, IL: Charles C. Thomas, 1972), and "Drug Abuse and Drug Policy," in *Acta Psych Scand.*, Suppl. 256 (Copenhagen: Munksgaard (1975).

2. The amphetamine epidemic in Japan after World War II is described by H. Brill and T. Hirose, "The Rise and Fall of a Methamphetamine Epidemic: Japan 1945–1955" (*Seminars in Psychiatry*, Vol. 1 (1969)), pp. 179–94.

3. Nobus Motohashi, *Addiction in Japan* (Toyko: Ministry of Health, 1973).

4. The opium epidemic in China is reported in I. L. Bird-Bishop, *The Yangtze Valley and Beyond* (London: John Murray, 1899), pp. 106–17, and Arthur Waley, *The Opium War through Chinese Eyes* (London: Allen & Unwin, 1958).

5. W. W. Willoughby, *Opium as an International Problem* (Baltimore, MD: Johns Hopkins University Press, 1930)'.

6. M. Heikal, *The Cairo Documents* (New York: Doubleday, 1973), pp. 306–7.

7. *An Australian Handbook on Drug Use* (Canberra: Australian Government Publishing Service, 1984).

8. *Ibid.*

9. Use and possession of less than 300 grams of marijuana was decriminalized in Spain in 1984 by the government of Philippe Gonzalez.

10. For an account of opiate addiction in the United Kingdom

see M. M. Glatt, "United Kingdom," p. 146 in *The Community's Response to Drug Use,* ed. S. Einstein (New York: Pergamon Press, 1980); and Nahas, *Keep Off the Grass,* 1984, pp. 265–8.

11. M. L. Harvey and J. C. Cross, *The Narcotic Officer's Notebook* (Springfield, IL: Charles Thomas, 1965).

12. F. Rosenthal, *The Herb Hashish versus Medieval Muslim Society* (Leiden: E. J. Brill, 1971).

13. Bird-Bishop and Waley.

14. *International Narcotic Control Board Annual Report* (Vienna: United Nations, 1989).

15. Carter, Parkerson, and Mamani, p. 159, in *Cocaine 1980* by F. R. Jeri. See note 4, Chapter 16.

16. "O you who believe, Wine and gambling are an abomination of Satan. Therefore avoid them that you may prosper." *The Koran,* Sura five verse 90.

17. Sully Ledermann, *Alcool, Alcoolisme et Alcoolisation* (Paris: Presses Universitaires de France, 1956).

18. G. G. Nahas, "The Ledermann Model Applied to the Frequency of Marijuana Use Among U.S. High School Seniors," pp. 485–90 in *Banbury Report II, Cold Spring Harbor Laboratory* (1982), and G. G. Nahas, "La Distribution de la Consommation des Drogues Toxicomanogènes d'après le modèle de Sully Ledermann" (*Bulletin Académie Nationale Médécine* 168 (1984): 195–201).

19. Paly, Jatlow, Van Dyke, Cabieses, and Byck, pp. 86–9. See note 1, Chapter 19.

20. "After 3 Years, Crack Plague in New York Only Gets Worse," *New York Times,* 20 Feb. 1989, p. 1.

21. Richard L. Berke, "Capital Offers a Ripe Market to Drug Dealers," *New York Times,* 28 March 1989, p. 1.

22. *The Economist,* 21 January 1989.

23. *Ibid.,* 8 April 1989, p. 54.

24. George F. Kennan, *Sketches from a Life* (New York: Pantheon Books, 1989).

Chapter 29   The Rehabilitation of the Cocaine Addict and the Will to Win the Cocaine Wars

1. Sandoz Rado (1890–1965). Psychoanalyst pupil of Freud. In 1931 he initiated the New York Psychoanalytical Institute of Columbia University. He reported his studies on

addiction in "Fighting Narcotic Bondage and Other Forms of Narcotic Disorder" (*Compr. Psychiat.* 4 (1963): 160).

2. Lowinson, pp. 346–54. See note 6, Chapter 13.

3. Nahas, Trouvé, and Maillet, "Prevention of Cardiotoxicity," pp. 1151–6.

4. Kleber and Gawin, "Cocaine Abuse," pp. 111–29.

5. Lewin, p. 87. See note 8, Chapter 8.

6. W. B. O'Brien and D. V. Biase, "The Therapeutic Community: The Family Approach to Therapy," pp. 303–16 in Lowinson.

7. DayTop Village, 54 W. 40th St., New York, NY 10018 (telephone 212-354-6000).

8. Phoenix House Foundation, 164 W. 74th St., New York, NY 10023 (telephone 212-595-5810).

9. Kids of Bergen County, P. O. Box 4407, River Edge, NJ 07661 (telephone 201-342-5437).

10. Straight, National Development & Training Center, 3001 Gaudy Blvd., P. O. Box 21686, St. Petersburg, FL 33742 (telephone 813-576-8929).

11. "Association Le Patriarche," Chateau de Lamothe, Saint-Cézert, 31530 Grenade-sur-Garonne, France (telephone 61-82-67-47).

12. On April 30, 1989, Monsignor W. B. O'Brien informed me that DayTop had a waiting list of 2000 cocaine addicts ready to start rehabilitation.

13. G. de Leon, "The Role of Rehabilitation," pp. 298–307 in Nahas, *Drug Abuse in the Modern World.*

14. Bejerot, *Drug Abuse and Drug Policy.*

15. G. Nahas, "The Other Asian Success Story: Drug Control," *Wall Street Journal,* 13 Feb. 1985.

16. I Corinthians 6:10.

17. Jeremiah 31:29; Ezekiel 18:2.

18. Imenhotep (fl. c. 2980–2950 B.C.). First physician to be recognized by his own name. He was also the architect of the Step Pyramid of Sakhara. He was deified as the Egyptian god of medicine.

19. Hippocrates of Cos (c. 460–377 B.C.). Greek physician, regarded as the father of medicine and physiology. He dissociated medicine from superstition and held that disease is caused by an imbalance of body fluids (humors) and that the body had to be treated as a whole. His high ethical and medical standards are commemorated to this day in the physicians' Hippocratic Oath.

20. Paré Ambroise (1510–1590). French surgeon who introduced life-saving techniques in the treatment of gunshot wounds.

21. Claude Bernard (see note 8, Ch. 28).

22. François Rabelais (c. 1494–1553). French physician, Renaissance humanist, and popular author.

23. Albert Schweitzer (1875–1964). Physician, theologian, philosopher, musicologist, organist, and a medical missionary in Lambarene, Gabon (Africa), for over 50 years, from 1913 until his death. He won the Nobel Peace Prize in 1952. His main books are *J. S. Bach, Quest of the Historical Jesus, Goethe,* and *Out of My Life and Thoughts.* He is one of the towering figures of the West in the 20th century.

24. A. M. Rosenthal, "Legalize Drugs? The Idea Deserves To Be Shot Down," *New York Times,* 24 March 1989.

25. On July 15–16 the seven most industrialized nations in the "West" (U.S., Japan, Germany, France, Great Britain, Italy, and Canada) held their tenth annual meeting in Paris. For the first time, their final resolution contained specific recommendations aimed at controlling the world epidemic of drug addiction, which, in their own words, "has reached dramatic dimensions." One of the recommendations mentions crop substitution for illicit plantations in the producing countries and with the help of the U.N., but it lacks the master plan with the financial and economic commitments required for an effective control of the cocaine traffic at its source. Other resolutions call for the convocation of two conferences in 1990 — one for reducing the demand for cocaine, the other for controlling the laundering of drug money by the banking system. Such recommendations address issues which are "downstream" and far removed from the main problem, which is left without a solution. To speak metaphorically, in order to control the production of wine one has to restrict the size of the vineyards, not the number of corks used in bottling the fermented grape juice. It is hoped that subsequent summit meetings will tackle, in a realistic fashion, the problem of controlling the production of cocaine and of other illicit drugs at their source.

Bibliography

Bejerot, Nils, *Addiction and Society*. Springfield, IL: Charles C. Thomas, 1970.

———, "A Comparison of the Effects of Cocaine and Synthetic Central Stimulants." *British Journal of Addiction* 65 (1970); 35–7.

Buck, Alfred A.; Sasaki, Tom T.; Hewitt, Jean J.; and Macrae, Anne A., "Coca Chewing and Health: An Epidemiological Study Among Residents of a Peruvian Village." *American Journal of Epidemiology* 88 (1968): 159–77.

Ciuffardi, Emilio N., "Contribucion a la quimica del cocaismo." *Revista de Farmacologia y Medicina Experimental* 2 (1949): 18–93.

Collier, H. O. J., "Drug Dependence: A Pharmacological Analysis." *British Journal of Addiction* 67 (1972): 277–86.

Cruz, Sanchez Guillermo, and Guillen, Angel, "Eliminacion de la cocaina en sujetos no habituados." *Revista de Farmacologia y Medicina Experimental* 2 (1949): 8–17.

Deneau, Gerald; Yanagita, Tomoji; and Seevers, M. H., "Self-administration of Psychoactive Substances by the Monkey." *Psychopharmacologia* 16 (1969): 30–48.

Drug Use in America: Problem in Perspective, 4 vols. Washington, D.C., National Commission on Marijuana and Drug Abuse, U. S. Government Printing Office, 1973.

Eddy, P.; Sabogal, H.; and Walden, S., *The Cocaine Wars*. New York: W. W. Norton, 1988.

Fabrega, Horacio, and Manning, Peter K., "Health Maintenance Among Peruvian Peasants." *Human Organization* 31 (1973): 243–56.

Fisher, S.; Raskin, A.; and Uhlenhuth, E. H., *Cocaine: Clinical and Biobehavioral Aspects*. New York: Oxford University Press, 1987.

Fleck, Ulrich, "Uber Cocainwirkung bei Stuporosen." *Zeitscrift für die gesamte Neurologie und Psychiatrie* 92 (1924): 84–118.

Freud, Sigmund, *Cocaine Papers*, ed. Robert Byck. New York: Stonehill, 1974.

———, *Cocaine Papers*, trans. S. Edminster and W. Hammond. Vienna: Dunquin Press, 1963.

Gay, George R.; Sheppard, Charles W.; Inaba, Darryl S.; and Newmeyer, John A., "An Old Girl: Flyin' Low, Dyin' Slow, Blinded by Snow: Cocaine in Perspective." *International Journal of the Addictions* 8 (1973): 1027-42.

Goddard, D.; deGoddard, S. N.; and Whitehead, P. C., "Social Factors Associated with Coca Use in the Andean Region." *International Journal of the Addictions* 4 (1969): 41-7.

Gold, M., *Cocaine 800.* New York: Bantam Books, 1984.

Grinspoon, L., and Bakalor, J. B., *Cocaine.* New York: Basic Books, 1975, pp. 1-308.

Gutierrez-Noriega, Carlos, "Acción de la Coca Sobre la Actividad Mental de Sujetos Habituados." *Revista de Medicina Experimental* 3 (1944): 1-18.

_____, "Alteraciones Mentales Producidas por la Coca." *Revista de Neuro-Psiquiatria* 10 (1947): 145-76.

_____, "El Cocaismo y la Alimentacion en el Peru." *Anales de la Facultad de Medicina* 31 (1948): 1-90.

_____, "Inhibicion del sistema nervioso central producida por intoxicacion cocainica cronica." *Revista de Farmacologia y Medicina Experimental* 21: (1949): 191-235.

_____ and Zapata Ortiz, Vincente, *Estudios sobre la Coca y la Cocaina en el Peru.* Lima: Ministerio de Education Publica, 1947.

Hanna, Joel M., "Coca Leaf Use in Southern Peru: Some Biosocial Aspects." *American Anthropologist* 76 (1974): 281-9.

Jacobi, August, "Die Psychische Wirkung des Cocains in ihrer Bedeutung fur die Psychopathologie." *Archiv für Psychiatrie und Nervenkranken* 79 (1927): 383-406.

Jacobson, Richard, and Zinberg, Norman E., *The Social Basis of Drug Abuse Prevention.* Washington, D.C.: Drug Abuse Council, 1975.

Jeri, F. R., *Cocaine 1980.* Proceedings of the International Seminar on Medical and Sociological Aspects of Coca and Cocaine. Lima, Peru: Pacific Press, 1980.

Jones, Ernest, *The Life and Work of Sigmund Freud,* in 3 vols. New York: Basic Books, 1953.

Laurie, Peter, *Drugs: Medical, Psychological, and Social Facts.* Baltimore, MD: Penguin Books, 1969.

Lewin, Ludwig, *Phantastica: Narcotic and Stimulant Drugs,* trans. from 2nd German ed. by P. H. A. Wirth. New York: Dutton, 1931.

Lindesmith, Alfred R., *The Addict and the Law.* New York: Vintage Press, 1965.

McLaughlin, Gerald T., "Cocaine: The History and Regulation of a Dangerous Drug." *Cornell Law Review* 57 (1973): 537-73.

Maier, Hans W., *Der Kokainismus* (Cocaine Addiction), ed. O. J. Kalant. English translation of 1926 edition (Leipzig: George Thieme). Toronto: Addiction Research Foundation, 1987.

Martin, Richard T., "The Role of Coca in the History, Religion, and

Medicine of South American Indians." *Economic Botany* 24 (1970): 422–38.

Mayer-Gross, W., "Selbstschilderung eines Cocainisten." *Zeitschrift fur die Gesamte Neurologie und Psychiatrie* 62 (1920): 222–33.

Mortimer, W. Golden, *Peru: History of Coca: "The Divine Plant" of the Incas with an Introductory Account of the Andean Indians of Today.* New York: J. H. Vail, 1901, repr. Berkeley, CA: And/Or Press, 1974).

Mule, S. J., and Brill, Henry (eds.), *Chemical and Biological Aspects of Drug Dependence.* Cleveland: CRC Press, 1972.

Murphy, H. B. M.; Rios, O.; and Negrete, J. C., "The Effects of Abstinence and Retraining on the Chewer of Coca-Leaf." *Bulletin on Narcotics* 21 (2) (1969): 41–7.

Musto, David F., *The American Disease: Origins of Narcotic Control.* New Haven: Yale University Press, 1973.

Nahas, Gabriel G., *Les Guerres de la Cocaïne.* Paris: France Empire, 1987.

———, "La Distribution de la Consommation des Drogues Toxicomanogènes d'après le Modèle de Sully Ledermann." *Bulletin Académie Nationale Médécine* 168 (1984): 195–201.

———; Frick, Henry C.; Gleaton, T.; Schuchard, K.; and Moulton, O., "A Drug Policy for Our Times." *Bulletin on Narcotics* 38 (1986): 3–14.

———; Trouvé, Renaud; and Maillet, Michel, "Prevention of the Cardiotoxicity of Cocaine by Nitrendipine, a Ca2 + Blocker." *Bulletin Académie Nationale Médécine* 169 (1985): 1151–6.

———; Trouvé, Renaud; Manger, William; Vinyard, Curt; and Goldberg, S., "Cocaine Cardiac Toxicity and Endogenous Catecholamines." In *Progress in Catecholamine Research,* ed. M. Sandler, A. Dahlstron, and R. H. Belmaker, Part B, pp. 457–62. New York: Alan Liss, 1988.

National Institute on Drug Abuse (NIDA) Research Monograph Series.

Clouet, D.; Ashgar, K.; and Brown, R. (eds.), No. 88: *Cocaine Abuse and Toxicity.* 1988.

Grabowski, J. (ed.), No. 50: *Cocaine: Pharmacology, Effects and Treatment of Abuse.* 1985.

Petersen, R. C., and Stillman, R. C. (eds.), No. 13: *Cocaine 1977.* 1978.

Superintendent of Documents, U. S. Government Printing Office, Washington, D.C. 20402.

Negrete, J. C., and Murphy, H. B. M., "Psychological Deficit in Chewers of Coca Leaf." *Bulletin on Narcotics* 19 (4) (1967): 11–7.

Offerman, Arno, "Uber die Zentrale Wirkung des Cocains und einiger neuen Ersatzpraparate." *Archiv für Psychiatrie* 76 (1926): 600–33.

Phillips, J. L., and R. W. Wynne, *Cocaine: The Mystique and the Reality.* New York: Avon Books. 1980.

Post, R. M., "Cocaine Psychoses: A Continuum Model." *American Journal of Psychiatry* 132 (1975): 225–31.

————; Kotin, J. K.; and Goodwin, F. K., "Effects of Cocaine in Depressed Patients." *American Journal of Psychiatry* 131 (1974): 511–17.

Redda, K. K.; Walkter, C. A.; and Barnett, G., *Cocaine, Marijuana, Designer Drugs: Chemistry, Pharmacology, and Behavior.* Boca Raton, FL: CRC Press, 1989.

Snyder, Solomon H., "Catecholanimes in the Brain as Mediators of Amphetamine Psychosis." *Archives of General Psychiatry* 27 (1972): 169–79.

Spitz, H. I., and Rosecan, J. S., *Cocaine Abuse: New Directions in Treatment and Research.* New York: Brunner/Mazel, 1987.

Stone, N.; Fromme, M.; and Kagan, D., *Cocaine: Seduction and Solution.* New York: Clarkson, N. Potter Inc., 1984.

Tatum, A. L., and Seevers, M. H., "Experimental Cocaine Addiction." *Journal of Pharmacology and Experimental Therapeutics* 36 (1929): 401–10.

Thornton, E. M., *Freud and Cocaine — The Freudian Fallacy.* London: Blond & Briggs, 1983.

Trouvé, Renaud, and Nahas, Gabriel, "Nitrendipine: An Antidote to Cardiac and Lethal Toxicity of Cocaine." *Proc. Soc. Exptl. Biol. Med.* 183 (1986): 392–7.

United Nations Economic and Social Council Report of the Commission of Inquiry on the Coca Leaf, Official Records, 5th year, 12th session, Special Supplement, Vol. 1, May 1950.

Uscategui Mendoza, Nestor, "Contribucion al estudio de la masticacion de las hojas de coca." *Revista Colombiana de Antropológia* 3 (1954): 207–89.

Von Scheidt, Jurgen, "Sigmund Freud und das Kokain." *Psyche* 27 (1973): 385–430.

Wittenborn, J. R.; Brill, Henry; Smith, Jean Paul; and Wittenborn, Sarah A. (eds), *Drugs and Youth: Proceedings of the Rutgers Symposium on Drug Abuse.* Springfield, IL: Charles C. Thomas, 1969.

Woodley, Richard A., *Dealer: Portrait of a Cocaine Merchant.* New York: Holt, Rinehart and Winston, 1971.

Yanagita, Tomoji, "An Experimental Framework for Evaluation of Dependence Liability of Various Types of Drugs on Monkeys." *Bulletin on Narcotics* 25 (4) (1973): 57–64.

Young, James Harvey, *The Toadstool Millionaires.* Princeton, NJ: Princeton University Press, 1961.

Index
Cocaine: The Great White Plague

A

L

M

N

O